The International Library of Psychology

THE SOCIAL LIFE IN THE
ANIMAL WORLD

Founded by C. K. Ogden

The International Library of Psychology

COMPARATIVE PSYCHOLOGY
In 4 Volumes

THE SOCIAL LIFE IN THE ANIMAL WORLD

F ALVERDES

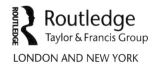

Routledge
Taylor & Francis Group

LONDON AND NEW YORK

First published in 1927
by Routledge, Trench, Trubner & Co., Ltd.

Published 1999, 2000 by Routledge
2 Park Square, Milton Park, Abingdon, Oxfordshire OX14 4RN
711 Third Avenue, New York, NY 10017

First issued in paperback 2015

Routledge is an imprint of the Taylor and Francis Group, an informa business

The publishers have made every effort to contact authors/copyright holders
of the works reprinted in the *International Library of Psychology*.
This has not been possible in every case, however, and we would
welcome correspondence from those individuals/companies
we have been unable to trace.

These reprints are taken from original copies of each book. In many cases
the condition of these originals is not perfect. The publisher has gone to
great lengths to ensure the quality of these reprints, but wishes to point
out that certain characteristics of the original copies will, of necessity, be
apparent in reprints thereof.

British Library Cataloguing in Publication Data
A CIP catalogue record for this book
is available from the British Library

The Social Life in the Animal World
ISBN 0415-20978-1
Comparative Psychology: 4 Volumes
ISBN 0415-21127-1
The International Library of Psychology: 204 Volumes
ISBN 0415-19132-7

ISBN 13: 978-0-415-75792-8 (pbk)
ISBN 13: 978-0-415-20978-6 (hbk)

CONTENTS

TRANSLATOR'S NOTE

I wish to express my very grateful thanks to my friend, Professor E. W. Patchett, for his invaluable help and advice in the work of translation.

K. C. Creasy.

PREFACE

THE aim of this essay is to present a particular chapter of Animal Sociology, in accordance with the most recent results of research in zoology and the psychology of animals. Animal Sociology has an important bearing upon Human Sociology ; for much that from an isolated standpoint seems to us purely human proves, in the light of animal and comparative sociology, to be typical of group psychology in general.

The subject is divided into Special and General Animal Sociology. So far as I am aware, a comprehensive survey of the latter is here attempted for the first time. In the special section, also, I believe that I frequently proceed along new lines. In the final chapter Human Sociology regarded from a biological standpoint receives such dis-cussion as the present state of comparative sociology permits.

F. A.

SOCIAL LIFE IN THE ANIMAL WORLD

I INTRODUCTION

Animal Sociology, or the study of the social life of animals, has already occupied the attention of a number of writers. Espinas was the first to write a comprehensive treatise on this subject ; others followed him, among them Doflein, Ziegler, and Deegener. One portion of the field has been particularly well surveyed, that, namely, which contains the so-called state-forming insects (bees, ants, termites, etc.), and excellent monographs have been written about them by Buttel-Reepen, Escherich, Forel, Wheeler, and others. But the scattered details of our knowledge of the social life of other animals have been much less carefully collated. Here, then, there is a gap to be filled.

Animal sociology has an important bearing on human sociology. As I have already mentioned in the preface, much that seems to us purely human, in the light of animal sociology comes to be recognized as typical of social psychology in general. The present treatise, however, is in no way concerned to show in how far much that we would call human is likewise found in animals, nor how much that we would call animal occurs in the behaviour of man (" Animal " as used here and later has, needless to say, no derogatory implications.)   Nevertheless, one of the

intentions of this essay is to show in what respects the social
life of men differs from, and in what respects it resembles,
that of animals. Comparison of the two will then enable
us to discover some of the basic instincts and impulses
upon which the whole edifice of human society is reared.
Researches such as these will form the task of a comparative
sociology of the future, and it is one of the main objects
of this work to collect the building stones for such a science.

A distinction can be drawn between special and general
animal sociology. The former is concerned with the different
types of social unit, such as the herd, marriage, the family,
and so on, while the task of the latter is to study those
general features which appear whenever any association is
formed, such as the establishment of a social scale, mutual
understanding, mutual assistance, etc.

While going through the literature of zoology from this
particular point of view, I realized how defective in many
ways our knowledge still remains. It is true that the subject
itself frequently offers very great difficulties. Lying in wait
for chances of observing the social life of the untamed
denizens of the woods, or the fish in the mountain stream,
requires much time and an ungrudging devotion to truth.
Numerous investigators have undertaken such tasks ; but
much remains to be done, and all those who come into
contact with animals : farmers, explorers, sportsmen, keepers,
and every animal lover, can lend valuable aid provided their
observations are judiciously made.

For my present purpose I have endeavoured to pay
special attention to all the most recent literature bearing
upon the subject. In addition, Brehm's work on the *Life*

of Animals was, naturally, a rich mine of information ; I
have made use of the fourth edition, edited by zur Strassen,
except where otherwise stated. I have also read a number of
travel books for the sake of what they might contain of
interest for animal sociology ; among these I should like
to single out that of von Schilling's, which, for this, as for
other purposes, has much to offer. Other books of travel,
which I will not name and have not quoted, often suffered
from the fact that the author thought it necessary to assume
a humorous tone whenever he was talking of animals or
natives. This procedure (which, as a rule, merely screens
the fact that the author has no positive contribution to make)
rendered the works in question useless for my purpose ;
for jokes, if we try to read a serious meaning into them,
often admit of so many interpretations that it is impossible
even to read between the lines.

The work of Köhler on anthropoid apes, and that of
Schjelderup-Ebbe on domestic fowl and wild ducks, proved
to be of the greatest importance for the chapter on general
animal sociology ; these investigations open up new paths
along which animal sociology may hope for great achievements. With regard to the exposition and interpretation
of facts, I sometimes differ not a little from earlier workers
in the field (especially Espinas and Deegener) ; but I have
done my best not to dwell upon these points of difference
so that mere controversy may not bulk too largely in the
following pages.

I have limited my theme in this work by confining my
treatment of animal sociology to the consideration of those
social creations in which animal psychology (i.e. a specific

social instinct) is the essential factor. Thus I have not discussed the phenomena of symbiosis, synoikia, parasitism, mimicry, hive-formation ; although I do not pretend that animal psychology plays absolutely no part in them. For information on these heads I refer to Balss, Buchner, Jordan, Jacobi, Doflein, etc.

Within the various agglomerations which animals are capable of forming, a distinction must be drawn between associations (mere collections) and societies (organic wholes). By associations I understand those chance gatherings produced solely by external factors (e.g. insects round a source of light). Societies, on the other hand, are genuine communities which exist in virtue of some particular social instinct in the animals concerned (e.g. the ant-state, a horde of monkeys). In short, no social instinct, no society ! (My definitions here differ from those of Deegener.) In the formation of an association the individual is guided by environmental factors, and not by other members of its own species ; a society, on the other hand, is formed when the individual is guided in the first place by the presence of others of its own species and only in the second place by environmental factors. In a genuine society, should need arise, the individual members will exchange a favourable environment for one less favourable, solely in order to satisfy a craving for companionship, and to remain in contact with other individuals.

Thus the social species among animals are those whose individual members possess a social instinct, while the solitary species are characterized by a lack of this instinct.

Whenever social beings are united by chance into an association (fowls in a fowl-run, school children in a class, recruits in a squad), manifold relations are quickly established, and the association becomes a society. Solitary beings, on the contrary, can only form associations, although on certain occasions a social instinct may be awakened within a solitary species and an association be thereby raised for a time to the level of a society (see below). Solitary life is certainly the more primitive manner of existence ; it is characteristic of all the lower forms of animal life, whereas societies are found only among the most highly developed species (cuttle-fish, insects, crabs, vertebrates). Social life, therefore, presupposes that mind and brain structure have both reached a certain level of development.

The question, which is the older, the family or the herd (the group, the society), and whether, perhaps, the one derives from the other, has long occupied sociologists. This statement of the question, as I shall show in detail, is altogether wrong ; the phylogenetic point of view is worthy of all respect, but it is possible to concede too much to it. For the genesis, on the one hand of mateship and the family, and on the other of the herd, depend upon two distinct principles, each of which has its own biological significance. These institutions cannot be derived from one another ; they stand side by side, and, among animals, sometimes they support and at other times they exclude one another. The situation is further complicated by the fact that marriage and the family obviously do not depend only upon the reproductive and the brooding instincts ; an additional element may be involved, namely a special instinct for mateship and for family companionship. This is proved by the case of those animals which propagate only during a special period of each year, and which yet live all their lives in company with their mates ; or whose family life is prolonged far beyond the time required to rear the young.

It may be stated at the outset that sexual relations among animals realize every conceivable possibility. Monogamy, polyandry, polygyny, whether mating be seasonal or permanent, are all to be found. Polyandry, however, is rare. Promiscuity also occurs ; it may be defined as that social state in which both male and female have intercourse with any number of individuals of the opposite sex taken at random. A distinction must be drawn between promiscuity as the normal state, and promiscuity as an accessory phenomenon. Given the second sense, then the existence of one or other of the two most common forms of mating (monogamy or polygyny) is the rule with the species in question, and only incidentally does one or other, or do both of the mates permit themselves to be unfaithful. Incidental promiscuity is by no means uncommon among animals (nor among human beings). But promiscuity as the normal relation of male to female, which would absolutely preclude any form of permanent mateship, is, on the other hand, by no means of such frequent occurrence among animals as some sociologists would have us believe. (Among human beings promiscuity is never the normal sex relation.) The permanent mateship of male and female is, nevertheless, a form of companionship which occurs only among the higher animals. I have consistently avoided the term

" polygamy " since it is so often understood to cover not only polyandry and polygyny, but, by some, promiscuity as well.

The term " instinct " has already been employed more than once in the preceding pages, and this is a suitable opportunity on which to explain briefly in what sense the term will be used in this book. As I have already dealt with this concept in a separate paper (1924) I shall now only add a few supplementary statements. Many writers speak of the instinctive and intelligent actions of men and animals as though these two types of action differed fundamentally from one another. As against this view, it must be asserted that a large instinctive element enters into every form of intellectual activity ; whilst no instinctive action ever runs its course altogether automatically and mechanically, but always contains in addition to its fixed and unchanging components a variable element more or less adapted to the particular situation.

Every act, A, is, therefore, at one and the same time a function of a constant, C, and a variable, V ; expressed as a formula this becomes $A = f(C, V)$. The constant is the instinctive element in the actions of men and animals ; the variable, on the other hand, is the element which produces in some cases an appropriate, in others an unforeseeable response to a situation. It must, of course, be emphasized that the analysis of the action A into the components V and C is a purely abstract analysis. V and C must not be taken as two more or less opposed natural agencies (as it were two souls) pulling the organism, now in this direction now in that, as they battle for supremacy ; they are merely symbols for two different aspects of the same reality. The difference between instinctive and intellectual activity is this, that in the former the constant, in the latter the variable predominates. In instinctive action then C is greater than V (C > V), in intelligent action C is less than V (C < V).

The purely instinctive, impulsive element in both instinctive and intelligent action is called the constant, for what is instinctive in every individual is determined by heredity. Neither animal nor man can transcend the limits of his native store of instincts. It is not alone the type of instinct which, for example, impels the insect larva just before the chrysalis stage to spin a complicated cocoon, characteristically different for each species, that justifies us in speaking of a constant. We have the same right to speak of a constant in the instinctive actions of the higher animals and man ; it is sufficient merely to mention those actions which are prompted by sexual and parental love, by the social and the egoistic instincts. But in a wider sense whatever man or animal does or leaves undone, has its roots in instinct, in impulse ; whatever is not potentially existent in this constant subsoil no power on earth can charm into being.

The variable factor contained in every act is most clearly visible in certain features of the behaviour of the higher vertebrates. Practice, experience, habit, also on occasion tradition—in short the whole past life of the individual— can greatly modify the course of subsequent behaviour. The reason is that in the intelligent activity of the higher animals V > C, whereas in any typical instinctive activity of insects, etc., V < C. In intelligent actions the variable produces on the one hand the suiting of the action to the given situation, and on the other hand its imprevisibility.

We have to postulate the existence of a variable not only in the intelligent actions of the higher vertebrates, but also throughout the whole of their instinctive activities. Take the case of a bird building a nest ; the variable appears in the way in which the individual bird sets about finding a suitable nesting place, and then, by means of purposeful and co-ordinated bodily movements, collects blades of grass, twigs, and floating feathers, and weaves them fittingly into the structure of the nest. This variable shows itself further in the greater skill displayed by the older birds in building. The acts performed in the operation of nest-building are by no means automatic, they are not mere " reflexes " ; neither are they purely intellectual (where V would be greater than C). On the contrary, genuine instinctive acts, in which C > V are everywhere involved. The fundamental impulse, C, invariably forms the constant basis which gives its " biological meaning " to the animal's whole procedure, and it is upon this foundation that all those individual purposive activities, which are determined by the variable V, repose. Exactly the same is true of the instinctive activities of insects, spiders, and so forth ; however rigidly and unalterably these may appear to proceed, in every case A = f (V, C).

In the majority of human actions V > C. But in the purely instinctive acts of insects, which are frequently executed with " intuitive " " somnambulistic " certainty without either practice or pattern, C often greatly preponderates. It is this that frequently renders the actions of insects incomprehensible to human beings. For much that in man is ruled by tradition and can be performed by the individual only after long practice, in animals is conditioned by instinct, and faultlessly executed at the first attempt. But we are, of course, still far from being able to say in each particular case of animal activity that here tradition (founded on V) is at work, and there instinct (K). This problem opens up a very wide field for future investigation

The notion of instinct defies all attempt to explain it ; for instinct, in common with other psychic attributes, came to be possessed by organisms in the same way as did their individual organs. Instinct is, so to speak, the " directions for the use of " the various organs. Why should the possession of directions for use be more mysterious, more inexplicable, than the possession of the tool to be used ? Instinct and organ are equally unexplainable.

In ordinary speech intellectual activity is called " conscious ", instinctive activity " unconscious ". On this point we must remark, however, that every act of man is attended with some degree of consciousness. This degree does not depend upon the relative amounts of V and C. It is just those acquired automatisms, which have nothing to do with genuinely instinctive acts (the daily winding up of one's watch, dressing and undressing) that are least consciously performed. As to the real nature of the consciousness of animals, we know nothing and can learn nothing.

Taking as our basis the formula $A = f (V, C)$, we realize that in human resolves, even in extreme cases, " emotional " and " rational " are not antitheses. C and V are involved in both, only in the first we have C > V, in the last V > C. For even a " rational " judgment depends largely upon the " emotional " organization and the mood of the moment ; its roots descend into depths beyond our penetration. On the other hand, in an action prompted purely by " feeling "— or by intuition—much is conditioned by the given situation and the given moment of time, and manifold experiences are interwoven with the " feeling ".

We are notoriously prone to give *post factum* a rational " explanation " of our impulses to act ; but these ultimately spring from the depths of the unknown and the unfathomable. That we so easily succeed in our " explanations " is due to our far-reaching adaptation to our environment (which we share with every organism) ; and we rarely become conscious of how many interpretations may usually be put upon our acts, nor of how easily we could find a whole bundle of motives for any one of them.

Because instincts are so restricted, so tied down, so limited in their scope, many irrational situations arise in the instinctive life of animals and man. We never, for instance, see ants, those wonderful architects, erecting a structure, however low, even when by this means they could bring within their reach an otherwise unattainable source of food. They try on the contrary every other method, only in the end to abandon their efforts if these are consistently unsuccessful. In the same way we see that although as social animals they are constantly assisting one another in all sorts of situations, ants never help each other to remove mites and other parasites from the surface of their bodies ;

this is left for each individual to do for itself, and in consequence many a parasite is left undestroyed. It would, of course, be easy to exterminate them entirely if the ants helped one another with the business.

Speaking quite generally, irrational situations arise whenever two instincts, which were they combined would produce a purposive whole (the permanent advantage of the individual or the species), remain independent of each other. But irrational situations also arise whenever two instincts, acting independently of each other, cause the individual to react in contradictory ways towards one and the same object. This can be observed not only in animals, but notoriously also in the case of human beings. In fact, absolute purposiveness is not found in any organism.

At the conclusion of this introduction let me mention, and dispose of a peculiar kind of error, namely that animals as opposed to men enjoy complete liberty of action, and therefore live in a paradise of untrammelled freedom. In sexual matters particularly an idyllic unconstrainedness is supposed to reign. The catchword of a romantic primitive condition has in this, as in other connexions, obtained widespread currency. All such talk is, however, founded upon fancy unsupported by fact. Some historian might find it a profitable task to investigate the origins of these and similar fantastic notions.

Primitive man, just as much as civilized man, has his own strong inward and outward ties and inhibitions beyond which he cannot go (Thurnwald) ; and the behaviour of an animal is determined in exactly the same way by the inner and outer restraints which are imposed upon it. Whosoever believes that sexual inhibitions do not exist for animals is on the wrong road altogether. Ideas such as these are frequently the result of observations carried out as occasion serves on apes and lions imprisoned in the cages of zoological gardens (cf. also Brehm, vol. xiii, p. 436). But is it permissible to draw conclusions applicable to the whole animal kingdom from the behaviour of a few separate individuals suffering more or less from claustraphobia? In other cases an observer is misled by watching the ways of dogs and other domestic animals, who, as a result of their association with human beings, have totally abandoned their normal social and sexual behaviour. Again, certain occurrences are wrongly interpreted, and a conclusion drawn from the behaviour of an animal in a single instance is applied in the first place to its behaviour in general, then to that of every animal of the same species, and afterwards, if possible, to animals in general.

The common notion that inhibitions first appear when the human stage in evolution is reached, and that they distinguish man from the " brute ", is without foundation. The specific characteristics of man are found in quite other spheres. " Brutes " in the evil and derogatory sense exist only in magination, not in fact. Men are fond of calling " brutes " those animals which, when trapped or hard pressed, turn and defend themselves. But " brutes " in the sense intended do not exist; what we do find are animals which act with great vigour both when defending themselves and in the pursuit of prey.

II ASSOCIATIONS

An association is formed by environmental factors causing a number of animals, whether of the same or of different species, to gather together in one place ; the mere presence of other animals does not keep the individual at the place in question ; it is, therefore, some factor in the environment which acts as the binding force. The aggregations of protozoa and small crustaceans which, under certain conditions, people in countless multitudes both fresh and salt water, are instances of associations ; so also are the collections of plant lice where the bond is merely a suitable feeding ground and not a social instinct. The gathering of birds and beasts of prey round the fallen body of a large wild animal in the tropics is an association, not a society ; as also are the gatherings of many species round a watering place in dry districts.

Groups of burying beetles (*Necrophorus*) gathered round the corpses of mice, lizards, birds, etc., are to be classed as associations. These beetles, alone or together, bury the dead body without themselves consuming any appreciable amount of it ; afterwards, however, it is invariably only a single pair of burying beetles that lays eggs therein, while the helpers, having done their work, withdraw ; thus the decaying corpse serves almost exclusively for the nourishment of the young which later emerge (Deegener, 1918,

p. 302). In burying beetles the burying instinct is invariably awakened by the sight of a corpse, whether the individual is alone or whether others are present ; each individual thereupon scrapes away at the task on its own account without any kind of mutual understanding with its fellow labourers. The effect of this instinct, which serves no useful purpose for the individual, but only for the offspring of the pair laying their eggs in the corpse, is of great importance in the preservation of the species.

Collections of ciliated infusoria at favourable points in their environment are further instances of associations. The slipper animalcule (*Paramœcium caudatum*) reacts positively to certain concentrations of CO_2 in water (Jennings, p. 100) ; the biological importance of this reaction is that it guides the Paramæcia to the aggregations of the bacteria which form their chief nourishment. Now Paramæcia themselves produce CO_2 ; it follows that in time ever-increasing " spontaneous collections " are formed where several Paramæcia have chanced to collect. There is, therefore, no question of a social instinct which brings Paramæcia together into one place, as used to be supposed. The mode of formation of this particular association gains interest from the fact that we have here an association formed, so to speak, in a self-created milieu.

A still further instance of associations is provided by the troops of migrating lemmings in the " lemming years ". The (probably unmated) males travel alone, each independently of all the others ; the female seldom migrates (Brehm, vol. xi, p. 265) ; only when a large number are migrating, or when external obstacles act as dams, do we get the impression of a gathering possessing the characteristics of a herd. The direction of the migration is determined by the given environment, so that, as a general rule, all the individuals travel in the same direction, even in different years.

III REPRODUCTION AMONG SOLITARY ANIMALS

The particular instinct which causes the members of social species to attach themselves to their own kind, or in the absence of these, to other animals, is wanting in the solitary species. Most of the lower animals lead a solitary life. If we disregard certain phenomena shortly to be mentioned, solitary animals never seek out other individuals. Speaking generally they exist, each one for itself, in extreme isolation, even when external conditions throw them together in no matter how great a number. Only at breeding time can we say that exceptions occur, in that the male and female then come together during the one sexual act, only to separate again immediately afterwards. In those species, however, where the fertilization of the eggs takes place without copulation there is not even an attempt on the part of male and female to come together.

Fertilization of the eggs without copulation on the part of the parents, that is to say without one particular male coming into actual physical contact with one particular female, occurs among many of the lower solitary animals ; it occurs among numerous Coelenterata and ringworms, among the lower snails and the majority of marine shell-fish, among *Echinodermata*, *Tunicata*, and many fishes (Meisenheimer, pp. 110–12). Eggs and sperm-cells are emitted into the water, and there fertilization follows. This emission takes place either without regard to the presence or absence of the other sex, or else individual members of the same species collect together beforehand in associations at definite places. In the latter case, whenever an individual discharges its sex substances this acts as a stimulus to the others, male and female alike. In many other species the male emits its sex substances into the water, and the sperm then penetrates into the female genitalia. In all these cases where a particular male does not enter into any direct relation with the female there can be no suggestion of the formation of a mateship.

Among the solitary species in which pairing and copulation occur, the individual may perform the sexual act either only once in its life, or repeatedly. The majority of insects pair only once (e.g. day-flies) ; spiders and some insects of the beetle, plant-louse, fly and butterfly classes, pair, as a rule, more than once. In general these repeated pairings take place promiscuously, that is to say the individuals copulate at random with members of the opposite sex. Here, there-fore, promiscuity is the general rule. In exceptional cases, however, among certain species of insects and spiders (see below) mateships may also be formed.

It is easy to show that promiscuity exists in the case of *Alytes obstetricans*. At each breeding season the female produces her eggs in three or four separate layings. These, as they emerge from the body of the mother, are fertilized by the male, and the latter immediately winds the whole laying, stringlike, round his hind legs. Thus it often happens that a male carries about, at one and the same time, strings of eggs belonging to several different females. In the case of the fish *Callionimus lyra*, which lives rather in associations than in societies, the male and the female deliver eggs and sperm while, with their abdomens pressed together, they rise to the surface of the water. Near the surface the fish, which appear to delight in copulation, separate, but after a short time go through the act again, sometimes with a different partner. Promiscuity also obtains among many reptiles.

True promiscuity occurs in the case of the cuckoo, which leads a solitary life throughout the year. In this species there are two males to every female. Each male remains in its own sharply circumscribed domain, and the females roam from one male to another, often pairing with six different males. It is altogether wrong to call this polyandry, for all the criteria of promiscuity are present.

IV SOCIAL INSTINCTS IN SOLITARY ANIMALS

Even among solitary animals phenomena of an undeniably social nature sometimes occur. On such occasions a social instinct awakens in them which does not manifest itself at other times. Thus groups of solitary animals are constituted for breeding, hibernating, migrating, and sleeping.

The swarms of dancing males formed by certain solitary insects, e.g. midges, flies, *Neuroptera*, day-flies, and *Perlidae*, are breeding societies. The females probably seek out these swarms, and as soon as a female approaches one of them, several males throw themselves upon her ; copulation ensues, however, with only one of the males. Among certain solitary insects, namely horseflies and some butterflies, the males and females collect in high-lying conspicuous places. Breeding societies are also found among certain species of snakes ; twenty or thirty individuals roll themselves into a kind of ball and remain thus for hours, performing, meanwhile, the sexual act, pair by pair.

Migrating troops are often formed by certain insects which normally live in solitude : by caterpillars, for instance, and the larvæ of other genera, by butterflies, dragon-flies, and locusts. Different species belonging to the same genus may combine to form a single migrating troop. Within these companies the striving of the animals concerned to hold together is unmistakable ; in consequence they travel over the ground or through the air in sharply defined masses.

The reason why these migrations take place is still unexplained ; they are not the result of a lack of food, or, at least, not always. Whenever, in hot weather, a number of locusts sit together in a compact group they become more and more excited until suddenly they take flight in a body. In their course they attract to themselves every member of their own species, so that the swarm increases like an avalanche (Brehm, vol. ii, p. 6). Thus what was originally an association becomes a society. In addition to these flying swarms of full-grown individuals, migrating swarms of locust larvæ occur. With dragon-flies the migrating host increases in the same way as with locusts, since every dragon-fly in the district traversed joins the throng.

The larvæ of *Sciara militaris*, a species of midge, lead, as a rule, a solitary life hidden in the ground ; at times, however, they come to the surface, collect in large swarms, and set out on migrations (hence the name army-worm). If one scatters the migrating insects they gather together again. In contrast to the animals that I have named, lemmings migrate as solitary animals, in the manner described above, even when they appear in large numbers.

Sleep societies occur among certain species of bees and wasps, as well as among butterflies (von Frisch, 1918, Schrottky). During the day the insects live apart, but in the evening the group in question always seeks out the same place ; the number of individuals present varies a little from day to day ; it may therefore be assumed that a few, at least, sometimes spend the night in one place and sometimes in another. Only males and unfertilized females are members of such sleep societies ; the fertilized females live in strict solitude, and devote themselves to the care of their young.

On certain occasions social tendencies generally manifest themselves among the males of some kinds of butterflies. Thus it is known that butterfly collectors can procure many males of these species by exposing here and there one or two males killed for the purpose. Other males then arrive and settle near them. But the assembled butterflies do not appear to enter into any discernible relation with one another.

Hibernating societies are found among various amphibians and reptiles ; thus in the autumn salamanders, slow worms, lizards, and snakes of the same species seek out common hiding places. But whether they are guided by a social instinct is as yet uncertain ; sometimes there can be no question of anything more than an association, since suitable hiding places are not very easily found. Hibernating societies also occur among certain solitary insects ; fleas, for instance, cluster together in buildings which are uninhabited during the winter.

In the case of amphibians it is impossible, according to Brehm (vol. iv, p. 26), to talk of a common social life ; the fact that they inhabit the same locality is the only bond between them. And yet frogs, for instance, are adapted for living in associations, and those companies of them which animate lakes and ponds, pools and rivers, during the warm months of the year may perhaps with some justification be regarded as intermediate between associations and societies. Frogs often begin and end their croaking all together, as anyone may hear for himself. The noise made by a frog in jumping into the water (the splash sound, Yerkes, 1903), the croaking, and the cry of a frog in pain acts as a warning to other frogs ; but no frog takes to flight before it has itself seen the enemy.   It is impossible to approach a frog in its native haunts if another nearby has already leapt into the water in flight.   Noises other than those mentioned have no sensitizing effect on a frog, though it may well have heard them.

V SPECIAL ANIMAL SOCIOLOGY : SOCIETIES

In this section we must discuss the sociological behaviour of those animals which, either temporarily or permanently, live a social life. I will endeavour in what follows to proceed with as little high-handedness as possible in dividing up my subject matter, making divisions only as they become necessary ; but since nature knows no scheme or system, a certain arbitrariness could not be avoided. It is not easy to delimit the concept of " temporarily social " animals from that of solitary animals displaying on occasion a social instinct. The last mentioned cases have already been discussed above. Among temporarily social species we will include those whose members consort with the opposite sex at least during a protracted breeding period, or which on other occasions as well seek members of their own or other species. The concept " protracted " is naturally a highly relative one ; how I understand it will appear in the course of my exposition. The term " permanently social animals " explains itself ; temporarily and permanently social species cannot be sharply divided from one another ; transitions of every kind occur. In order to divide the " states " of bees, ants, termites, etc., suitably from all other animal societies (for on account of the morphological and psychological differentiation of their " castes " these " states " are formations of an altogether special kind), I shall in the first instance discriminate between (A) species in which every individual normally attains full sexual development, and (B) species in which the greater number, or the vast majority, of individuals are asexual, i.e. the " state " forming insects.

A SPECIES IN WHICH EVERY NORMAL INDIVIDUAL BECOMES CAPABLE OF REPRODUCTION

Among the species all of whose members, apart from abnormalities, are capable of reproduction, we may divide those in which reproduction takes place at fixed seasons from those which breed practically without interruption. The majority of social species are included in the first category ; among them rutting periods alternate, in regular yearly rotation, with periods of sexual inactivity. The second category possesses a peculiar interest in that it includes human beings.

For members of the seasonal species breeding time brings with it a more or less radical change in all their habits. Individuals which, until that time have led a solitary life, then attach themselves to partners of their own race ; or, again, companies of animals which have been living peacefully together break up into separate couples and families ; at the very least a radical reorganization of the herd occurs. In what follows, therefore, we shall have to consider (1) the behaviour of both temporarily and permanently social animals during breeding time separately from (2) their behaviour at other periods. Those species whose members live permanently mated are relatively least affected by the seasonal rutting period ; yet even in their case this period brings with it manifold changes in the daily conduct of their lives.

1 Reproduction

In considering behaviour during reproduction we must distinguish between (*a*1) relations to the other sex, and (*a*2) relations to offspring. The case (*a*3) of those excluded from reproduction deserves separate attention.

*a*1 *Relations to the Other Sex*

Sexual intercourse among social animals with seasonal rutting periods may take place either (*b*1) by the members gathering together and emitting their sex substances into the water, as we have already seen to be the habit of some solitary animals living in associations ; in this case there is no mateship and no formation of a family. Or (*b*2) by each animal entering into separate sexual relations with another.

*b*1 *The Emission, in common, of the Sex Substances by the Collected Individuals*

The majority of fishes, especially the salt-water species, emit eggs and sperm loose into the water ; fertilization is then left to chance. In this connexion the species which most interest us are those which live in swarms ; among them it is common for the females to swim above the males during spawning so that the eggs as they sink must pass through water saturated with semen (Brehm).

*b*2 *Individual Sexual Relations*

Sexual intercourse between one individual and another may either take place (*c*1) promiscuously, or (*c*2) a mateship may be formed between two members of opposite sexes. Either such mateships are strictly adhered to by both mates, or again both may adopt promiscuity. In that case promiscuity as an accessory phenomenon stands side by side with permanent mateships as the rule. If one or both of the parents remain for a time with the offspring then the mateship gives rise to the family ; but many parents forsake the eggs before the young emerge.

cI *Promiscuity as the General Rule*

We met with promiscuity as the normal form of sexual intercourse among solitary animals, insects in particular ; further among fishes, amphibians and reptiles, and in the case of the cuckoo. Promiscuity among gregarious animals is extremely rare. Formerly people were inclined to take it for granted that within a herd the sexual act is performed indiscriminately between the individual members (for a time this was quite wrongly supposed to be the custom among primitive races). It was imagined that if at breeding time any male came together with any female within the herd copulation at once ensued.

Some species of lizards living gregariously adopt promiscuity. True promiscuity appears to exist among bats which live gregariously ; in any case several males have been observed to pair, one after another, with the same female ; other males which happened to be present at the same time exhibited complete indifference. Promiscuity is said to have ruled among North American bisons ; but this assertion must remain a matter of controversy. The North American cow-bird (*Molothrus ater*), which lives gregariously throughout the year, is promiscuous in its habits ; it is interesting that this bird, like our cuckoo, is a parasite so far as hatching out the eggs is concerned. Promiscuity very probably exists among black game and capercaillies. While the domestic cock, as is well known, keeps his hens together throughout the year, among the two last mentioned species, during pairing time the male forsakes immediately after each copulation the females which had collected at the pairing ground. Capercaillies have, on an average, four, and black cock eight hens. Apart from the short periods during which they meet every day at the pairing ground, the sexes, in this case, lead a perfectly separate life (Doflein, p. 473). A polygynous mateship is not formed, as it is among certain other gallinaceous birds ; and it is quite possible that individual hens seek out the pairing ground now of one male and now of another. Over and above this there are black cock that fly from pairing ground to pairing ground, fighting there with other males for the favour of the female. According to Naumann (vol. viii, p. 264) pairing takes place promiscuously among ruffs (*Machetes pugnax*), which live in societies.

Promiscuity is asserted to exist among argus-eyed pheasants, quails, and also among hares. But perhaps permanent partnerships are the rule here too, and their existence is overlooked by observers only because the partners do not abide by them over-strictly. Promiscuous habits were long ascribed to foxes, but it has now been established that they live monogamously (Brehm). The fact that house dogs pair promiscuously is a consequence of their domestication, seeing that the special conditions of their association with men prevent any permanent mateship.

It has never been ascertained whether polygynous mating

takes place among wild pigs in the breeding season or whether promiscuity is the rule. The latter is frequently asserted. At breeding time the males, which otherwise keep to themselves either alone or in separate herds, unite with the herds of the females, these latter being accompanied by the sexually undeveloped young. Long-drawn-out battles then take place among the males, which result either in the removal of a rival by one of the males, or the mutual toleration by two equally strong males of one another's presence within the same herd. In this last instance it is conceivable that promiscuous pairing ensues (it might be permissible to speak of some kind of " group mating " here), or, again, the right of possession over the different females may have been strictly delimited as between the rivals.

The greater number of fishes emit eggs and sperm into the water without the male and female thereby entering into any individual relations with one another. This; however, is not always the case ; among perch and other species, the female lays its eggs and several males then discharge their sperm over them. If the females lay eggs more than once during one and the same period of sexual activity, then promiscuity and not polyandry exists.

Sticklebacks and *Gobius* belong to the fishes which live in swarms, males and females together, except during the pairing season. At the beginning of the breeding period the males isolate themselves, and each one then builds a nest within a circumscribed area which is thenceforth stoutly defended against every intruder. When the nest is finished the male fetches some female, which thereupon lays a few eggs in it. The male then fertilizes the eggs. On the next and following days the male again regularly fetches another female, until a considerable number of eggs has been deposited. The females in this way lay their eggs in the nests of different males.

c2   Mateships

As against promiscuity we may contrast mateships. These may be monogamous, polygynous, or polyandrous ; the last is rare. Mateships are either (d1) seasonal, that is to say the partnership is dissolved at the end of the rutting season, or they are (d1) permanent or enduring mateships, when they outlast the periods of sexual inactivity which recur each year ; among many birds of which seasonal reproduction is characteristic, the monogamous mateship, once concluded, lasts throughout life until death separates the mates. Mateships are either solitary, in which case the male separates himself and his mate, or his harem, from others of his own kind, or several mateships (whether monogamous or polygamous) join together to form a community. Permutations and combinations of these different possibilities yield several categories. Unfortunately our knowledge is still very imperfect ; thus in respect of certain species we do not know whether they live in seasonal or in permanent mateships. Such doubtful cases will be mentioned later in their appropriate connexions.

d1   Seasonal Mateships

Seasonal mateships do not outlast the breeding period, this owing to the fact that members of the species concerned live a year at most, or that, in the case of animals living longer than a year, a new partner is chosen at the beginning of each breeding period. Seasonal mateships may be either ($e1$) solitary, or ($e2$) within the herd.

$e1$ Solitary Seasonal Mateships

In solitary seasonal mateships the partners, linked together in ($f1$), monogamy, ($f2$) polygyny, or ($f3$) polyandry, live for the time a solitary existence, and do not enter into relations with others of their own kind.

$f1$ Monogamy

Monogamous solitary seasonal mating is found among a number of beetles.   In these species male and female remain together throughout a summer, copulation taking place several times; the couples live, at most, in associations, not in societies. Only in the case of a very few insects does the life of the individual, after it is full grown, last more than a year (Korschelt); it is, therefore, perfectly justifiable, wherever mateships are formed, to speak of seasonal mating. In the case of the dung beetle (*Minotaurus typhoeus*) the method of forming a mateship is for the female to choose one out of a number of males ; she always knows him again, and keeps by his side (Doflein). The lamellicron beetle (*Ateuchus sacer*) lives paired with a mate within an association formed near a favourable feeding ground. Male and female co-operate in making their pills of dung, and these they defend against other members of their own species, later using the pills as food for themselves or their offspring. Among wood-boring *Passalidæ* and other beetles, the monogamous parents feed the larvæ and guard the chrysalides.

The male and female of water spiders (*Argyroneta*) remain together throughout the year ; also certain species of crabs live together in pairs (Doflein, p. 467). Whether among water spiders and the crab species in question the case is one of seasonal or permanent mateships has not yet been determined.

Seasonal mating occurs among certain fish species. Thus the female salmon lays its eggs and they are then fertilized at intervals by the male which remains present whilst they are being laid (Brehm). Rivals are driven off by the male. During the fights which occasionally arise it sometimes happens that young males arrive and fertilize the eggs ; these play the part of *tertii gaudentes*, as young deer do in similar circumstances (accessory promiscuity). If the full-grown male meets his death, the female fetches another to the spawning ground (second mateship). It is inadmissible to regard this as polyandry. Societies formed by shoals of small carp (*Rhodeus amarus*) break up at pairing time into monogamous partnerships, only to collect together again after the time is over. Graylings (*Thymallus*) consort together in pairs during the breeding season. Among *Labrus* and some *Cichlidæ* both parents protect the eggs and supply the young with food.

In many amphibious species the couples seem to cling to one another at pairing time with great affection ; however, they separate at the close of the breeding period (Brehm).

Rhinoderma, for instance, live monogamously. The female lays eggs repeatedly, one or two at a time, at intervals which may extend to several days, and after their fertilization by the male collects them into a gular sac,

Some reptiles live in pairs during the breeding season ; cobras, *Cyclura*, wall lizards (Doflein, p. 468), also emerald lizards and pearl lizards usually live together in pairs throughout the breeding season (permanent mateship ?).

With some birds the mateships do not outlast the breeding season ; so that a fresh mateship is entered into with a different individual at the beginning of each such period. Some mammalian beasts of prey live monogamously but none throughout life. In certain cat and marten species the two sexes consort with one another both during and after the breeding period in order to protect and nourish the young. In the case of lions a fresh mate is chosen at every rutting time ; during pairing time monogamy is the rule. Male and female jaguars live together monogamously for four or five weeks ; during the rest of the year they lead a solitary life. Foxes live monogamously ; the female accepts only one suitor and the father (contrary to earlier belief) defends the young and brings them food. Wolves live in couples during the spring and in packs during the winter. Wolves, foxes, and bears live mated for a certain period even after the actual rutting time is over (Doflein, p. 479).

It is uncertain whether seasonal or permanent mating is the rule among certain other mammals. These appear in couples throughout the year, and are accompanied for a time by their young. The species concerned include certain kinds of dolphins, *Sirenoidei*, pigs, deer, and antelope, also apparently the blue whale. It seems very likely that for some of these species, especially the small antelope, permanent mateship is the rule.

Our ignorance about the duration of some animal mateships is in part due to the fact that we have not yet any exact information about the rutting times and laying periods of many kinds of tropical wild animals. The reason for this is that the majority of hunters sally forth with a purely sporting interest, i.e. they aim at the destruction of a large amount of game in the shortest possible time. Unfortunately the only method known to the majority of men of dealing with the animal creation, in so far as it is not a question of purely domestic animals, is that of shooting them down or in other ways doing them to death. According to Berger, the assumption that African wild beasts breed throughout the year is false ; on the contrary, breeding time falls, generally speaking, in the dry season ; but this differs in different regions. The length of the period of gestation varies with the species ; and, correspondingly, the rutting time varies from species to species. Animals kept in confinement naturally do not afford a reliable source of information in consequence of their completely altered external conditions. In opposition to Berger, Schuster believes, amongst other things, that at least in the case of certain antelope species, no periodic heat occurs, and that consequently the breeding period extends over the whole year. (With regard to zebras and rhinoceros see below.)

f2   Polygyny

Seasonal solitary polygynous mateships exist among some bark beetles. The male establishes a sort of nuptial chamber under the bark, one after another a number of females enter it, and each after the resulting fecundation gnaws out a hatching place in which she lays her eggs.

Many mammals, too, live in such mateships. The following behaviour is typical of many species : outside pairing time the males do not concern themselves with the females, but live an independent life, either singly or in troops. When mating time arrives they seek out the females and either attach themselves to the troops of the latter or collect together the largest number of females they can, and fight every rival. Only young males incapable as yet of reproduction are tolerated. Among Indian buffalo the herds break up at the commencement of pairing time into small bands, each gathered round one steer. In the following remarks bands of females, guarded by a single male, and sometimes accompanied by other immature young males, will be described, for the sake of shortness, as " harems ". It is characteristic of the seasonal harem that it is abandoned by its overlord every year at the end of the breeding period. The harem either scatters to the winds (e.g. among elks) or remains together as a " herd of mothers ". It should be stated in regard to the organization of a seasonal solitary harem, that in certain cases the leadership of the herd is taken over by the male overlord ; on the other hand this business is often left to an old and experienced female who also presides over it during the period of sexual inactivity, when the male has long since taken himself off.

Among stags at rutting time the strongest male drives off all younger males and rivals from the herd of females, comprising from six to twelve animals, which he has selected. The herd is invariably led by a female, and all the other females follow her guidance. This leadership obtains even during rutting time. During the vigorous battles between the principal stags, the younger males sometimes stealthily enter the herd and cover its female members ; they likewise appear when the old males have become impotent, and then themselves cover the females (the two last-mentioned instances should be rated as accessory promiscuity). Sexual activity takes a similar course among other deer, among many antelopes, among wild sheep and wild goats.

Among Indian elephants, moufflon and waterbuck the harem also possesses a female leader. The function of the accompanying male is then merely to possess the females. In earlier times such a harem of elephants consisted of thirty or forty full-grown females ; that to-day much smaller harems are encountered is due to the severe persecution which elephants have suffered during the last few decades. We find solitary harems among most deer, among many antelopes, among wild goats and wild sheep, without it being possible, up to now, to establish with certainty whether in every case the male or the female takes the lead. The information we at present possess is to some extent self-contradictory. Among gaur, a species of Indian wild buffalo, every herd of from eight to ten head contains, outside rutting time, two herd bulls. At pairing time an otherwise solitary bull joins the herd, who proves himself more than a match for the herd bulls and rules unrestrained as long as the rut lasts. In spite of his presence, the herd bulls usually remain with the herd.

Wild cock pheasants seem to live monogamously and the male takes a share in the rearing of the young ; on the other hand, half-domesticated pheasants are polygynous, and the male, in this instance, does not concern himself with his

offspring ; when his sexual instincts are satisfied he thus
forsakes the harem which he has gathered ; the females
scatter and devote themselves, each independently of the
others, to the care of their young. The behaviour of black
game and capercaillies at dancing time apparently lies on
the borderline between polygyny and promiscuity, as
we saw above.

f3   Polyandry

Polyandry is rare (Deegener, p. 258) ; it occurs, so far as I
was able to see, only as a form of solitary seasonal mateship,
and so should be treated in this context. It is invariably
connected with the fact that in the species concerned the
males are considerably smaller than the females. Among
Alcippe, a cirripod belonging to the race of crabs, the females
live as a rule in associations ; from three to twelve dwarfish
males join a female and remain with her through life. In
the case of the worm *Bonellia* up to eighteen males attach
themselves to every female ; here, likewise, the males are
disproportionately small compared with the females.
Polyandry also exists among certain spiders, where two
males attach themselves to each female and copulate
repeatedly.

e2   Seasonal Mateships within the Herd

The different types of seasonal solitary mateships have
been discussed in the previous section ; such mateships
occur when a monogamous couple, which have united for
one breeding period only, or when the polygynium or the
polyandrium remains solitary. There are, however, cases
in which the individuals united in a seasonal mateship

remain members of a larger herd unit. In these instances the
herd of sexually inactive animals undergoes a reorganization
at the beginning of the sexual period ; it does not, however,
disperse into separate partnerships, on the contrary these
continue to keep together. Those seasonal mateships united
into a larger unit are either (*f*1) monogamous, or (*f*2)
polygynous ; no case of polyandry has ever been known.

*f*1 *Monogamy*

From the nature of the case it is frequently very difficult
to decide whether the mateships of gregarious animals are
seasonal or permanent, when the animals in question are
monogamous and yet do not abandon their communal
life during the breeding period.   To get unimpeachable
results one would have to mark paired animals in some
way which leaves them unharmed and then watch them
carefully from year to year.

Many rodents which construct their burrows colony-
fashion, and which obviously have dealings with one another
inside these stationary societies, have been found at breeding
time in their burrowing places in pairs, e.g. marmots, rabbits,
prairie dogs, chinchillas, beavers, and rats.   Since rabbits
are now said to live in mateships that last several years, it
may be conjectured that this also occurs in the case of one
or other of the above-named rodents.   The oryx antelope
(Doflein) and many whales live monogamously within
wandering herd groups. The Beluga whales live in this way
in schools within which the animals live in pairs, accompanied sometimes by a young one.   Steller's sea-cows
(*Rhytina stelleri*), which in their time inhabited the Behring

Sea, and are now extinct, lived monogamously within the herd unit. Their discoverer, Steller, reports that a male came two days in succession to the beach where the female, which had been killed, was lying (Brehm). Further, the sea-otter (*Latax*) lives monogamously in a herd unit ; male, female, and the young which belong to them keep together within the group. In all these cases, as I have already remarked, it is not certain whether we should speak of seasonal or permanent mateship ; were the latter proved true in one or other case, then the species concerned would have to be classified not here, but under a heading to be discussed later.

Many birds, as is well known, nest in colonies. Thus they do not abandon their gregarious mode of life even during the time of incubation ; it is above all a social instinct, not the specially favourable nature of the environment, that forces them together. It is often doubtful whether we have here a case of seasonal or permanent mateship. But since the majority of birds live in mateships we will leave all bird colonies to be considered together in their appropriate place ; let it suffice, at this point, to hint that perhaps one day the existence of seasonal mateships among one or other of the bird species which hatch in colonies, will be established beyond doubt. Among Central European swallows, which nest in colonies, the couple remain together often during one incubation only, pairing afresh for the next.

*f*2 *Polygyny*

The cases in which seasonal polygyny occurs together with the continued existence of the herd as a unit are easier to establish. The structure of a herd of sexually active animals differs considerably from that of a herd during the asexual period. At the period of sexual inactivity the sexes not infrequently divide into separate groups, or at least hold together in two distinct bodies within the herd. The awakening of the sexual impulse brings about a complete alteration in so far as the herd now consists entirely of harems. Let us take seals as an example. In the species *Callorhinus*, the fur-yielding seal, the bulls live separately in herds in the open sea, and so, to a certain extent, do the bachelors, i.e. the males which have not reached pairing age ; these bachelors also appear sometimes to attach themselves to the herds of females with their young. At the beginning of the breeding season the old bulls are the first to come to land, where they occupy their accustomed rocks ; later the troops of females appear, and immediately the males begin to collect together harems, numbering usually from fifteen to twenty-five, and at the most forty, females (Doflein, see illustration, pp. 475–8). The females may be either about to be delivered, or if one year old only, still virgin. Furious fights then take place between the males until gradually a balance of power is established and the rights of each animal are defined and recognized. The old bulls, defeated in combat and driven off, and the bachelors prevented from pairing by the lords of the harems, hold themselves in two separate groups. When all the cows have been covered the harems are dissolved and all the animals betake themselves again to the open sea. Reproduction follows precisely the same course among other species of seals.

d2 Permanent Mateships

What serves to characterize a permanent mateship is the fact that the partners hold together either through several breeding periods or for the whole of their lives. Permanent mateships may be either monogamous or polygynous. Polyandrous partnerships, which could be described as forms of permanent mateship, are so far unknown. Both monogamous and polygynous mateships may be either (e1) solitary or (e2) comprised within more or less extensive herd communities. Permanent monogamous mateships occur both among species with uninterrupted, as well as among those with periodic reproductive activity. The latter case is especially noteworthy because among species with regularly interrupted sexual activity it cannot be the sexual impulse alone which holds the monogamous couples together throughout the year ; as I have already said in the introduction, a second instinct is necessary before a true mateship can be formed.

e1   Solitary Permanent Mateships

f1   Monogamy

Monogamous solitary permanent mateships are characteristic of many bird species. The common raven and numberless birds of prey live in solitary couples throughout the year, and do not migrate to more temperate zones during the winter. Other birds of prey and also partridges do not migrate, and while being strictly monogamous (mating in some cases, like the partridge, for life) gather together into flocks during the winter. On the other hand grebes live permanently in solitary couples which migrate together to the south, and together come back again.   Other birds, on the contrary, travel in flocks to warmer regions, although the couples not uncommonly remain united within the flock.

Among chaffinches returning from their winter quarters, males and females fly in separate flocks, the males about a fortnight ahead of the females ; the divided couples usually meet one another again at the old hatching ground, each bird there rediscovering its old mate.   In some parts the males remain behind throughout the year while the females only migrate, so that in such cases the monogamous mateship outlasts even a winterlong separation of the mates. In many species the couples, on their return, seek out the same spots, if not the same nests.

Permanent mateship, among some species, does not last a lifetime ; among others, on the contrary, it is terminated only by the death of one of the mates.   In many bird species lively battles are fought between the males for possession of the females ; and in the case of species which commonly pair for life it may happen that an unfavourable issue costs the defeated bird his mate (*Haliaëtus*).   In some species the female vigorously supports her mate in battle with a rival.   Sometimes the mates are greatly attached to one another ; thus, if old nightingales, which have paired beforehand, are imprisoned, they regularly die ; whereas younger birds, which have not paired, can endure captivity (Brehm). Widowed birds pair again, both in a wild state and in captivity if suitable mates are available.   Among storks, and some birds of prey, if one partner perishes the survivor is said to seek out a new mate so that with the help of the latter it may complete the rearing of the young (Doflein).

Among other species of birds, on the contrary, one parent alone brings up its offspring ; whilst in yet other species the father, at least, cannot do this unaided.

Monogamy is either strictly observed (cranes, geese, and swans), or one of the two mates permits himself an occasional infidelity (accessory promiscuity). Cases have been known in which a female stork, already paired, has allowed itself to be trodden by a strange male. Coots live monogamously, and the couples hold together apart from other birds during the period of incubation, though an unmated hen may lead the male into a passing infidelity. Contrary to what used to be asserted, and in contrast to related species found in South America, the African ostrich is monogamous (Brehm). The male arranges the nest, and male and female relieve one another during incubation. As there are more females than males, the surplus hens wander about and allow themselves to be mounted by males which have already paired ; these females, since they do not arrange a nest for themselves, lay their eggs in any nest they come across ; thereupon, a battle with the rightful owner may take place over the nest, in the course of which all the eggs may possibly be destroyed. Outside pairing time ostriches live gregariously ; how long the mateships last has not yet been ascertained.

There are many mammals of which we cannot yet say whether their solitary monogamous mateships are seasonal or permanent. Solitary permanent mateships seem, at least, to occur among the various species of rhinoceros ; the same applies to some apes, and their hybrids. According to Volz, the orang-utan lives in solitary permanent mateship.

The permanent mateships of the rhinoceros are possibly

connected with the fact that, according to Schuster, these animals breed uninterruptedly throughout the year. Deeg., it is true, asserts that in this case, too, breeding is periodic. In the same way permanent mateships among apes are rendered more probable by the fact that, for some species at least, it is firmly established that the males never lose their reproductive powers, and that the females menstruate at monthly intervals throughout the year. But even in these cases the impulse, already alluded to, prompting the formation of a real mateship should not be altogether lost sight of.

f2   Polygyny

The domestic fowl provides a typical instance of solitary and permanent polygynous mateship, since the cock keeps his hens together throughout the year. In the case of the Nandu, the South American ostrich, the cock bird lives during breeding time with a flock of hens, numbering from five to seven, inside an area which he holds throughout the period against every other member of his own species. The hens lay all their eggs together in one nest, but incubation is done by the male alone. During the time of incubation the hens remain together within the area held by the cock bird. First of all the chicks alone follow the father, and the hens join them later on. When hatching time is past several polygynous families, with the chicks belonging to them, collect together in larger groups ; nevertheless whereas the family tie holds fast beyond the breeding period, the tie which holds the larger union together is looser, for the separate families attach themselves now to one and now to another flock. During breeding time then, the Nandu lives in solitary polygynous mateships, and these mateships are permanent because they continue in existence during the period of sexual inactivity when the birds congregate together with the members of other family units.

Among mammals each herd of guanacos and vicunas consists, both during and after breeding time, of a number of females and one male ; only young males as yet sexually undeveloped are tolerated by the old male. The latter leads the harem, looks after its safety, and covers its retreat. If the male is killed, the females, left leaderless, wander about aimlessly.

Among primitive Asiatic wild horses each herd consists of a stallion and his harem, which contains from five to fifteen mares. Herds of zebras are organized in the same way ; if the stallion perishes the mares are received into another harem (Schillings). Several herds of zebras, each made up of a stallion and his harem, may temporarily unite into larger herds (see below) ; such groups are, nevertheless, but loosely connected, and break up easily into their component parts, the separate polygynous mateships. During these temporary alliances each stallion watches jealously over his harem. Among zebras there is no settled time for parturition ; Deeg. has observed coverings to take place and foals to be born at all times of the year.

Where, as in South America, the domesticated horse lives in a semi-wild state, every stallion is given from twelve to eighteen mares which he holds together. Each group lives apart, and keeps to itself, and should the groups, by any chance, merge with one another, e.g. as the result of a large number of horses being driven together, the various troops immediately separate out again. The surplus stallions are gelded, and these geldings keep apart in herds of their own. All stallions, even those which hitherto have passed their lives in a stable, show the instinct to collect together a number of mares and possess them (Brehm, vol. 12, p. 699), and the latter offer no resistance ; clearly then both mares and stallions possess an instinct for such polygynous mateships.

Among one of the Asiatic species of wild asses, the herd leader is likewise a male ; and the older he becomes the more mares he gathers about him, the number varying from three to fifty. If the male is killed, the herd breaks up. With the Nubian wild ass, on the contrary, it is said that the herd, which contains from ten to fifteen mares, is led by an old mare (Brehm) ; such a harem, however, is always the property of a single male, who obstinately defends his rights.

Every herd of kangaroos frequents a special grazing place, and sometimes more than one, these being linked by well trodden pathways. One and the same herd remains a constant unit and does not mingle with others. Each is led by an old male which it follows blindly, either when grazing or when in flight. When pairing time begins, the leader claims the females belonging to his herd as his own property, but the claim is not allowed without fierce battles with other males who have come to maturity since the previous breeding period. These battles may result in the breaking up of one herd into several, which thereafter exist as separate units, each led by a male.

Solitary and permanent polygynous mateships also occur

among some apes, e.g. among macaques ; the horde forming the harem is always led by a male, and contains from ten to fifty animals. Some writers have called this leader " the pacha ". He suffers no other male near him, and any rebellious animal is disciplined with kicks and cuffs. In climbing, the members of the horde are careful to keep to the route taken by the leader, and the whole procession then goes through identical movements at any given place. If the leader is killed the herd becomes completely helpless. According to the authorities on this subject, each such herd is believed to consist of the ramifications of a single family ; and the leader is claimed as its founder ; this, of course, is merely an hypothesis. During the search for food, the leader keeps guard, and in case of need warns the herd, which thereupon takes to flight. During the retreat the leader, from time to time, looks back at the pursuer. Each horde usually clings to a special area, which it never abandons. If two hordes encounter one another the leaders sometimes fight a duel, and if one is mortally wounded his harem may well join in the fray. Brehm reports that occasionally one horde will attack another and drive it from its dwelling place (which, in India, is sometimes an ancient temple).

e2 *Permanent Mateships within a Herd*

Permanent mateships within a larger unit are of special interest since human marriages must be classified under this heading. Among animals such mateships may be either ($f1$) monogamous or ($f2$) polygynous, and the same is true of men.

*f*ɪ   *Monogamy*

I shall discuss the subject of permanent monogamous mateships within a herd in special detail because sociologists insist that such mateships are unknown in the animal kingdom, and "therefore" conclude that, as found among men, they are purely arbitrary institutions having no " natural " foundation. This is one of the numerous cases where zoology is called in, quite wrongly, to corroborate some purely fictitious assertion.

According to the interesting facts ascertained by Reichenow, the gorilla comes under this heading. The West African gorilla lives in bands numbering from ten to twenty, the East African in bands numbering from twenty to thirty animals. During the day the herd scatters over a fairly wide tract of country, but reassembles in the evening. Each gorilla builds a nest for the night, those of the full grown animals measuring from two to three metres across. From the arrangement of the nests relatively to one another, Reichenow was able to arrive at important conclusions about the family life of gorillas. In the virgin forests of Northern Africa the nests are built on the ground ; only females with very young offspring build their nests about one and a half metres above the ground. In the south, on the contrary, the females and the younger animals alone build nests, and these are placed from five to six metres up in the trees ; the males spend the night on the ground without a nest at all. Apes belonging to the central region seem to occupy a middle position, since in their case some members of a herd will build a nest near the ground, and others one from three to five metres above it. A shelter against rain is never provided. The nest is used always for one night only, and in the morning, on departure, is not infrequently befouled with excrement. According to Reichenow, nest-building probably depends entirely upon tradition, and not upon a sharply defined and specialized instinct (as among birds), for only gorillas captured after a certain age show, in captivity, any inclination towards arranging a bed, a thing never found when the animals are taken very young from their mothers. Perhaps, then, a difference in tradition is responsible for the fact that gorillas build differently in the north and in the south. Köhler, however, in the course of his investigations with chimpanzees, came to the conclusion that nest building among this species is purely instinctive (see below).

According to Reichenow (p. 16), the gorilla lives not polygynously, but monogamously within its hordes (this contradicts Zenker's assertions) ; the sexes do not associate merely during each breeding period, but remain together during many years. The half-grown apes evidently stay for a long time with their parents, perhaps even until they found a family of their own. The horde therefore consists of a number of monogamous couples and their offspring. It is not known in what family relationship the members of a horde stand to one another. Reichenow observed that a horde is never composed of more than five families. This division into families is expressed even in the daily arrangement of the nests. Reichenow found that in the northern region the nests of a horde were arranged not irregularly, side by side, but in ordered groups, which were divided by spaces from eight to fifteen metres wide. Each group contained two large nests, those namely of the two parent apes, and from one to two smaller nests belonging to their half-grown offspring, who from the age of about three or four years onward occupy sleeping places of their own. As long as the young are still quite small they spend the night with the mother, who builds a specially soft nest placed specially high.

Von Kappenfels (quoted by Brehm) describes the father as forcing his mate and his offspring to pluck and fetch fruit for him, dealing out boxes on the ears when this is not done quickly and lavishly enough ; Zenker relates the same thing.

Very old male gorillas, and these alone, live without a mate. According to Reichenow, they are always animals which have ceased to have any desire for the female, and which have lost touch with their companions in consequence of the break up of their families ; whether an old male is expelled by one or more of the younger males is not known. Such occurrences—still hypothetical as far as apes are concerned—play a part, as is known, in discussions of the " Oedipus complex ". We have likewise no information as to the fate of old females living independently of a mate within the herd ; they are not met with living apart from other animals of their own kind.

The chimpanzee, like the gorilla, lives in bands, and the former avoids the latter ; Reichenow believes that inter-breeding between the two species is therefore very improbable, for every female is protected by her own horde. It is unanimously denied by travellers that old gorillas carry off women. Reichenow is of the opinion that these

tales of woman-stealing gorillas originated in the notion
that sorcerers could assume the forms of gorillas, leopards,
or elephants, and in this guise were able to play all sorts of
tricks upon their fellow creatures. Like the gorilla the
chimpanzee builds itself a sleeping nest every night, which
it uses only once ; this is built in the trees, twenty to thirty
feet above ground. What has been said of the nest-building
impulse of gorillas is true also of chimpanzees ; according
to Reichenow this depends upon tradition, according to
Köhler it is purely instinctive. The chimpanzee knows
how to protect itself against rain with branches, which it
lays over its back. Much less is known about the family
life of the chimpanzee than about that of the gorilla. The
former are encountered in hordes of twenty to thirty head.
According to Reichenow, since material suitable for observation is entirely lacking, assertions about polygyny among
chimpanzees are purely imaginary. Very old chimpanzees
live quite alone without a mate.

Every horde of gorillas or of chimpanzees inhabits a
perfectly well-defined and limited area, whose size is
regulated according to the number of animals in the horde ;
for a horde of average size its diameter, according to
Reichenow, measures about fifteen kilometres ; the domain
of an old male, living alone, is correspondingly smaller.
These in particular defend their area obstinately against
every intruder. The hordes wander through the whole
domain in every direction, and in so doing the animals
contrive never to spend two successive nights in the same
place, although at the end of several weeks they ever and
again return to the neighbourhood of a former sleeping

place. This wandering life is conditioned by the vegetarian habits of gorillas and chimpanzees, who, in their wild state, feed exclusively upon fresh shoots. Unlike gorillas, a horde of chimpanzees seems always to travel in unbroken file, one member following close on another. These circumstances produce a constant coming and going in any region where chimpanzees abound.

Other species of apes also live monogamously within a horde ; this seems to apply, for instance, to the members of the *Callithrix* family, which inhabit South America. In this instance, the female bears from one to three young at a birth, and carries them about with her ; from time to time she induces the male to carry the children, which he does without hesitation. Tame guinea pigs live monogamously within their herds. Their breeding period lasts throughout the whole year ; at the beginning two unmated males may fight for an unmated female ; one of them pairs with the female, and from then on this ownership remains undisturbed. Among Patagonian cavy (*Dolichotis*), a species allied to the guinea pig, which lives in herds, the mates are so closely attached to one another that they come together again even if they are separated for months and the female is shut up with another male (Brehm). Wild rabbits construct their burrows in the form of colonies where the different passages in which they live communicate with one another. They have been said to form monogamous mateships which last for several years ; the male, nevertheless, is believed to indulge in accessory promiscuity, seeing that he copulates occasionally with unmated females. Further investigation of rodents living in colonies will perhaps result in the discovery of other species among which monogamous mateships last for several years.

Permanent monogamous mateships within a community probably occur among many of those birds which brood gregariously. Penguins, herons, wild guinea fowl, some species of sand-pipers, sea-gulls, sea-swallows, auks, guillemots, parrots, bee-eaters, swifts, certain birds of prey (e.g. the majority of the vulture species), ravens, starlings, some thrushes, the weaver bird, many doves, ducks, cormorants, all are gregarious throughout the year, and live in monogamous unions which, among many of the species named, probably last for several years, if not for life. Thus all species of parrots, so far as is known, live in strict monogamy throughout their lives. If one of the mates is shot the other (e.g. among araras) not infrequently allows itself to be caught. Herons in their brooding colonies are also strictly monogamous, and the same applies to the flocks of penguins which collect at brooding time, often numbering hundreds of thousands. In some colonies different species may possibly brood side by side (as do different species of vultures). Among many kinds of birds, even in large flocks, a pair of mates may be recognized by their devotion to one another's society. At brooding time too, birds which brood in colonies generally set out together, in large or small groups, on the quest for food, as anybody may observe, for himself, each year in the case of starlings. Rose-coloured starlings are monogamous, and nest gregariously. During the day the male feeds the brooding female ; at night the latter remains on the eggs, while the males depart together for a sleeping place which is perhaps several kilometres away. Sparrows are also monogamous and brood gregariously, and while the female broods the male from time to time betakes himself to the society of other males.

It used to be supposed that button quails (*Turnices*) lived polygynously; this has proved to be erroneous, they are monogamous. Moreover among them, as among phalarope, the females are larger and more brilliantly coloured than the males; here only the females dance and fight for the possession of the males, while the latter alone hatch the eggs.

Among the penguins already mentioned, at breeding time the brooding colonies, which sometimes contain members of more than one species, are traversed by innumerable pathways cutting each other at right angles. Each of the rectangles thus formed is taken possession of by a pair of penguins, and here the nest is built, either below, or on the level of, the ground. Nests below ground level are connected with each other by similar paths. Endless quarrels occur over the nesting place and the quadrangular space which surrounds it. The nest itself is made of collected pebbles, which the birds occasionally steal from one another. Murphy has described the gregarious life of the guano birds of the Peruvian coast; most instructive photographs show the birds brooding, flying together, and engaged in other activities.

In the case of the small green black-capped parrot, as many as twelve pairs build their globular nests so close together as to give the impression of a solid mass of twigs; each nest, however, has its own entrance and its own outer room and brooding chamber. The sociable gros-beak

(*Philetaerus socius*) nests, colony-fashion, in trees. Each pair builds and roofs its own nest, but the nests are so closely packed together that they resemble a single structure with a roof above, and innumerable entrances below. Each nest is used only once ; at the next brooding time the new nests are fastened underneath the old ones, so that the structure grows larger and larger, until, at length, it crashes to the ground.

House pigeons live and nest gregariously ; as pigeon-fanciers know by experience, from four to eight pairs at least must be kept at the same time, otherwise the birds fly away and join some other flock. In certain species, according to Whitman, the sexes do not recognize one another at first sight, but only by their behaviour ; homo-sexual inclinations and actions occur with males and females. Once mated the female pigeon is usually faithful ; this is less true of the male ; all the same, even if he does occasion-ally visit other unmated females, he is so far faithful to his mate that he assists in the preparation of the nest, relieves her regularly during the breeding period, and feeds the nestlings. The infidelity of the male may, then, be claimed as a case of accessory promiscuity. The male recovers from the loss of its mate much more quickly than the female. If the fancier attempts forcibly to re-mate the birds, they often go back to their original mate on the first opportunity. Nevertheless it would seem that among pigeons mateships are not life-long, but last only over a number of brooding periods.

Schjelderup-Ebbe has made a number of most important observations on the life, after mating, of gregarious wild ducks.   One female never attempts to decoy a mallard belonging to another.   During the selection of mates the male approaches the female ; but the latter does the choosing, that is to say she either avoids the approaching male or accepts his advances.   If she accepts him a monogamous union is formed ; if she does not the male turns his attention to other unmated females until his wooing meets with success.   No hen bird ever allows herself to be forced into mating with a mallard.   The superiority of one suitor over another does not influence the female in her choice.   According to Schjelderup-Ebbe both male and female are strictly faithful to one another.   Unmated males are always eager to waylay already mated females.   If the mate is stronger than the new-comer he tries to drive off the latter ; but in spite of this the intruder sometimes succeeds in treading the female, for once he is in the " pairing trance " no biting or pinching on the part of the rightful mate has any effect.   If the new-comer is stronger, the dispossessed mallard does not dare to defend his partner, but merely sets up a loud outcry.   (According to Schjelderup-Ebbe, the respective superiority and inferiority of one bird to another in a bird community is always perfectly well known to its members ; see below under " pecking order ".) When the hen bird begins to brood the mallard, according to Brehm, leaves her, and joins with other drakes to form special flocks, or even mates again with a second hen bird which has remained unmated.   But when the ducklings have reached a certain age, the mallard again joins the female and her brood.   The mergus often nests in colonies ; in this case two hen birds, even if they belong to two different species, not infrequently lay their eggs in one nest, brood in common, and share the work of feeding and caring for the young without making any distinction between their own and the other's offspring. Among a species of weaver bird (*Munia malabarica*) two couples often share a common nest in which both the hen birds lay their eggs and hatch them out. Supplementary mention may be made of the Brazilian anis (*Crotophaga ani*). Some half-dozen of the hen birds build a common nest and also carry out the incubation of the eggs in common, two or three birds sitting on the nest simultaneously, and being relieved from time to time by other mothers. But since I could not, from the literature on this subject, make sure of the exact nature of the mating habits of this species, I merely quote these facts for what they are worth.

ƒ2 Polygyny

The tarpan, the primitive European wild horse, now extinct, lived in herds numbering several hundred head. Each of these herds was sub-divided into a number of families, each family consisting of a stallion and several mares ; no stallion allowed younger stallions capable of reproduction, nor even an older rival within his harem. The stallions often carried off domesticated mares, and on this account the South Russian peasants used to lay traps for them. Among zebras, and South American horses reverted to their wild state, several stallions and their harems may join together into more or less loosely organized communities ; but even in this case the property rights of each stallion are strictly respected.

Some authors have given highly imaginative accounts

of those ape societies which are composed of several permanent polygynous mateships. On the basis of the information at present available, the organization of such a horde
may be portrayed somewhat as follows. Among polygynous
species any ape-herd of considerable size consists of several
harems. By definition, every harem is composed of several
females with their offspring and a number of half-grown
males and females, held together by a full-grown male
(called by these authors " the pacha "). The first care of
every male is his own large family ; he looks after its safety,
and makes sure that his more or less numerous wives remain
true to him (Brehm, vol. 13, p. 575). Those of the latter
who commit an act of infidelity are cuffed and pulled about
by the " pacha ". In these polygynous families it seems
that only the females, not the males, carry the young about.
Several families, each led by its " pacha ", join together to
form larger bands ; the leaders then make it their common
task to guard the horde, in which they may relieve one
another. The defence of the horde against external enemies
is undertaken by all the " pachas " together. Since in every
herd of apes constant quarrelling is the general rule, dis-
sensions may also arise between these leaders. Each
band lays claim to a special area. At night the apes usually
huddle close together and keep one another warm.

Contrary to a widely accepted belief, all serious writers
agree that promiscuity is never the general rule in a horde
of apes ; promiscuity as an accessory phenomenon does,
however, occur. Let me seize this occasion to emphasize once
again that apes do not deserve the imputation of abnormal
sensuality (Brehm). Adult males retain their reproductive

powers throughout the year, and the female menstruates every month ; this, and the protracted helplessness of the young, certainly contribute to hold such polygynous mateships together. Baboons, especially, live in groups led by several " pachas ", each accompanied by his harem (Schillings, 1905, p. 393), and this is probably true of howling monkeys (*Myetes*) as well. But even in this species, a " pacha " and his harem occasionally form an independent family. Hordes composed of different species of long-tailed monkeys are not rare. But even when every member of such a group follows the same leader, it is, nevertheless, certain that he does not lay claim to every female in his horde. In spite of the fact that only one such leader is present, given a sufficient number of individuals, here again a number of polygynous mateships may be formed within the horde. Now there are also hordes of monkeys all of whom belong to the same species, which are led by one ape alone, even though the horde contains several other full-grown males. So far as I could gather from the literature on the subject, it is supposed that, in these hordes, the leader claims all the females for himself. It is, however, possible that, as with a horde composed of different species, the " chief " possesses his own particular harem within the horde, and that the same applies to each of the other males. A further possibility, not to be summarily rejected, is that the stronger male, but he alone, may encroach with impunity upon the harems of the weaker, just as among ducks, according to Schjelderup-Ebbe, only the stronger treads the mate of a weaker one without meeting with opposition on the part of the admitted owner. All these are obscure points where monkeys are concerned ; it is very much to be desired that some light should be shed upon them.

a2   Relations between Parents and Offspring : Families

A family may arise out of a mateship, but this does not necessarily happen. Many animals, even those which unite in seasonal monogamous mateships (fishes, amphibians, reptiles), abandon the eggs after they have been laid, and concern themselves no further with them. A distinction may be drawn between (b1) parent families, (b2) father families, and (b3) mother families, to accord with the cases in which both parents, or only the father or the mother, remain with the offspring. If the young are abandoned by both parents, whilst remaining united among themselves for a time, they may be said to form (b4) a child family. When one or both of the parents guard the eggs, but not the young after they are hatched, we have a preliminary stage of family formation. Among many species the fostering of the brood is a complicated matter. The families may be seasonal or perennial according to the period required by the young for development.

b1   Parent Families

Parent families occur among *passalides* and other wood-boring beetles, where the parents feed the larvæ, and watch over the chrysalis. Both male and female of the fish species (*Eupomotis*) guard the nest built to contain the eggs ; the young, after they are hatched, return to the nest every evening for three weeks, and both the father and the mother keep watch over them (Doflein, p. 587). It is not impossible that in this case the example of the parents teaches the young to seek for food and avoid danger. Similarly among *Labrus*, and some *Cichlides*, both parents provide for and protect the eggs and young.

The parent family is also very common among birds and mammals. With monogamous birds the female usually builds the nest while the male only carries the material. Among weaver birds the male alone does the building, the female helps, at most, in the fitting out of the nest. Nest-building depends not on tradition and instruction but on a highly specialized instinct ; for young birds construct a nest at the fitting season without ever having seen one before. The only difference made by practice is that the older birds build more cunningly than the younger. Generally speaking the nest serves only to shelter the brood, but with tits both the parent birds and their young often spend the night in it, even in winter.

The cock bird relieves the hen during incubation ; often he brings her food. In many species both parents feed the offspring, and not infrequently carry away their excrement.

The parental instinct in birds is so strong that it is easy to foist eggs or nestlings not too obviously different from their own upon a couple to whom they do not belong. Substitutions of this kind even occur in nature ; half-fledged nestlings which have lost their parents will sometimes fly to a strange nest, possibly that of another species, and are there fed, together with the nestlings already present, by the parents of the latter. It is well known that the hen cuckoo lays her eggs in the nests of other birds and practically never broods herself. The fact that cuckoos' eggs found in the nests of hedge-sparrows, water-wagtails, etc., always in the same degree resemble those of these species, depends, according to Rensch, upon the fact that the owner throws all too dissimilar eggs out of the nest. Thus the cuckoo trades upon the parental instincts of the birds whose nests it invades. The newly hatched and still sightless cuckoo ejects the offspring of its foster parents from the nest with movements of its wings and back, but in spite of this the parent birds invariably look after the interloper until it is fully fledged. Thus we have the following anomaly : the singing-birds worry the full-grown cuckoo just as they do other enemies, e.g. birds of prey and owls, by emitting piercing screams when the female cuckoo approaches their nests, whereas their all-powerful parental instinct prompts them invariably to tolerate the egg or tend the young bird left with them. A South American duck (*Metopiana*) lays its eggs, like the cuckoo, in the nests of other birds, namely in those of coots, sea-gulls, etc., and never, apparently, builds a nest of its own.

If one of a pair of brooding birds dies the survivor often brings up the brood alone. But the males of many birds of prey cannot do this. With house pigeons, if one mate perishes whilst brooding the other very soon desists from the task. The parent birds of some species (ostriches, peewits, corn-crakes, larks, partridges, ducks, etc.) entice an enemy away from the nest by a cunning retreat, pretending to be wounded, limping, etc.

If the hen bird lays a second batch of eggs, the cock very often assumes entire charge of the first brood. Young swallows share with their parents the task of feeding the second brood (Groos, p. 12 ; Brehm).

When the young birds are fledged they are taught flying and other accomplishments. Often the old birds perform flight movements in sight of the nestlings, entice them oue of the nest by dangling food in front of them, or push them over the edge of the nest and catch them again, if necessary, in mid-air. Crested divers take their chicks down with them when they dive, tucked under their wings. As soon as young wall swifts are able to leave the nest the parent birds may be seen flying with them through the streets of our towns, uttering piercing cries ; by this means they are taught to fly and catch insects. Male and female falcons teach their young to capture prey. One parent on the wing drops the prey, and the young must catch it in full flight ; if they miss it the other parent, flying under them, catches it before it touches the ground, carries it up again and lets it fall once more from above the young birds. These exercises serve also as practice in flying, the young birds imitating the example of their parents.

When nestlings are full grown the parents very often drive them from the nest, on the other hand they may remain under the protection of the parents even until the second year, as happens in the case of some ducks. The parent gray goose cannot fly, consequently the young do not migrate in the autumn, but remain with the old birds during the winter (Doflein, p. 692). The male partridge at first guards his family alone ; later, however, when the young males are suffieiently developed, they take it in turn to keep watch over the brood.

Among polygynous birds the care of the young usually devolves upon the female, but in the case of the Nandu it is undertaken by the male.

Among many mammals the father helps in protecting and instructing the young ; it is probably in the nature of things that the male of a monogamous species takes a greater interest in the young than the male of a polygynous species. In those mammal species where development is especially show two or more litters may remain under the care of their parents at one and the same time.

Among some beasts of prey the father lives for a time with the mother and the offspring. Thus the male lion is said to help in the procuring of food, and to defend both its mate and its offspring. Some beasts of prey, while they are still young, learn how to hunt under the guidance of their parents ; in the case of lions this period of instruction is said to last a year and a half. Male foxes, contrary to earlier views, also defend their mate and their offspring. On the other hand it is uncertain whether the male wolf helps in the rearing of the young.

Among monogamous *Ungulata* (wart-hogs, certain red deer, antelopes, gazelles etc.) the male helps to defend and instruct the young. In respect of wild rabbits we have two contradictory assertions, namely that the father protects the young and the mother hides them from him ; perhaps it is a case of the habit varying with the district. Among *Ungulata* living in polygynous permanent families the male leader always protects the whole harem, including the young.

With both polygynous and monogamous apes the father

guards the young ; often the mother, as far as is possible, keeps the offspring away from the father ; in the case of *Callithrix*, however, we saw that the female sometimes induces the male to relieve her, temporarily, of her burden, which he does willingly. In certain ape species, when kept in captivity, the father assumes the care of the young on the death of the mother (Brehm, vol. 13, p. 561). Proof that apes are by no means sexually unrestrained is to be found in the fact that the male of a polygynous species may care for his female alone once she has become a mother, and for her offspring, taking thenceforward no notice of other females (Brehm, vol. 13, p. 591). The mother chimpanzee carries her young about until their third year. The first attempts at walking alone are prompted by the mother placing the infant on the ground, whereupon it utters piercing cries and immediately runs back to her. But the mother puts the frightened infant down again and again, until at last it gains courage to crawl a few paces. According to von Allesch, the mother chimpanzee teaches her offspring to crawl in the third month ; standing opposite to it she holds it by one paw and forces it to follow her on three legs while she goes backwards ; or she puts it down beside her and leads it stumbling along. Orang-utan females kept in captivity have been observed to teach their offspring to eat bread by chewing it before them. Pfungst never observed that the females of other ape species teach their young, as they are commonly asserted to do. According to him, too, games between the young and the old are always started by the young. Yerkes mentions that mother apes will sometimes carry about a still-born infant for more than a

F

month, until all that remains of it is an unrecognizable shred
of skin.

b2   Father Families

When the father alone takes charge of the young, a father
family is formed. In a certain sense such a family may
be said to have been formed when the father guards the
eggs after they have been laid, even though he takes no
further trouble over the offspring when they are hatched,
as occurs in the case of the grass frog. The male of *Alytes
obstetricans* carries the eggs about with him in a long string
wound round his hind legs until the larvæ emerge, and
defends these strings against marauders ; but the larvæ
are left to themselves. In contrast to this the male *Rhinoderma* not only carries the eggs in his gular sac but the young
as well, until their metamorphosis is complete, while
among some other frog species the tadpoles are carried about
on the back of the male.

The male stickleback builds a nest and induces a number of
females to lay their eggs in it, in the way described above.
If his nest is taken from him he suffers himself to be pursued
and ill-treated by others of his own species, but as soon as
his nest is returned to him he immediately puts all his
assailants to flight, and returns to the defence of his nest
again (Deegener, p. 237). His psychic condition strongly
affects his bodily appearance ; when thus dispirited, he pales,
though normally at pairing times his body is a bright
scarlet. Not only the eggs but also the young, after they
have hatched out, are guarded and kept together by the
father ; runaways are swallowed and brought back to the
nest. It is probable that young fish, forsaken by the father,

attach themselves to families still led by the male parent. A few other fish species may be named ; the male *Protopterus* defends his offspring as long as they remain in the nest ; the male *Macropodus* and that of allied species seizes in its mouth young which have strayed from their foam nest and brings them back to shelter ; the male of *Arius* carries both eggs and young for a time in its mouth, and later on, if danger threatens, hides them there again ; the male *Amia* leads its family of young for four months.

b3 *Mother Families*

It is more frequently the mother than the father who, unassisted, guards the young. The females of some species of leeches carry their offspring about for a time ; the young attach themselves to the body of the mother with their suckers, and if detached, always return to her. The female of certain species of bugs guard their eggs and their young. The female earwig (*Forficula*) guards eggs and young in a hole which she digs herself, and collects them together again if they get scattered. The female mole-cricket (*Gryllotalpa*) digs a hole for its eggs and guards them and, for some time, the young as well, although this does not prevent her from gradually devouring a certain number of the latter (cannibalism is, indeed, of very common occurrence in the animal world, see below). With many arthropods, specially among crayfish, but also among spiders, the mother carries the eggs about with her ; in the case of spiders the mother may even guard the young. Among *Lycosidæ* and scorpions the young take refuge on the mother's back. The female scorpion is said actually to catch prey and tear it into pieces for its young. In the case of *Copris*, a dung beetle, the female remains with the larvæ during their metamorphosis, and is even supposed to assist them to emerge from the chrysalis. The female of some species of cuttlefish (octopus and other allied species) watches over the eggs, and passes a constant current of water over them from her funnel.

Mother families also occur among fishes. The female of Heterotis lays her eggs in a nest and later leads the swarm of young. Among some species of *Cichlidæ* the female carries the eggs and the young in its gullet ; the young afterwards swim near the mother, and when in danger collect round her head, or are sought out, one by one, and sucked into her throat again.

The female marsupial frog carries its eggs in a pocket on its back until the young tadpoles emerge. The female pipa toad carries its young in a pouch of skin on its back until their metamorphosis is completed. Female crocodiles watch over their eggs, help the young to emerge, and lead them to the water. The female alligator protects its young even after this point. Female pythons guard their eggs ; whether they also protect their young is not known.

Mother families are the rule among polygynous birds (except in the case of the Nandu). Chickens, for instance, learn from their mothers how to avoid danger, how to pick up food (Morgan), and (according to other writers) their peculiar method of drinking.

In the case of the feline beasts of prey the mother drags small living, or half-dead animals up to her young, provided that the father does not also take his share in rearing them (see above). Among the majority of beasts of prey one of the chief cares of the mother is to keep the father away from the offspring to prevent him from devouring them. She sets free her prey in the presence of the young, and by catching it they prepare themselves for future predatory exploits. Later on the mother takes her offspring with her on her hunting expeditions, and it is only when they have themselves mastered the art that they leave her. Such instruction may require months, for though the predatory instinct is innate, it is perfected only by teaching. Young foxes are taught by the mother in a similar fashion. Female polar bears and seals carry their young to the water and teach them to swim. Solitary mother families are found among some of the *Ungulata* (e.g. among elks). Where the larger gregarious mammals are much pursued, the herds may sometimes split up into mother families. Thus Schillings (1905, p. 128) repeatedly saw herds of elephants consisting of a mother and six or seven younger animals of different sizes, very probably all of them children of the old female born in the course of the previous thirty or forty years.

A " mother herd " is formed when a number of mothers and their offspring unite into a society without the fathers (see below).

b4 *Child Families*

If the children only, without their parents, unite and form a society, a " child family " or brotherhood is the result. Processionary caterpillars, and other species of the genus *Thaumatopœa*, which have emerged from the same

mass of eggs, remain together permanently. In their migrations they form the well-known " processions ".   One caterpillar leads the way, after it two or three others, and then
the rank and file in threes and fours.   The insects creep along
in an unbroken chain, and if this chain is ruptured at any
point the alarm thus created may spread to the leaders,
and the procession comes to a standstill until the broken
connexion is re-established.   Deegener is, in my opinion,
quite wrong in calling such a gathering an association and
not a society, giving as his reason that " no positive
advantages can be proved to result from it " (1918, p. 86).

   Hyponomeuta caterpillars build a common dwelling nest.
If scattered, they strive, according to Deegener, to reunite
and build another, whereby various different " child
families ", i.e. the offspring of different parents, mingle
without hesitation, even when there is a considerable
difference in their ages.   Small bands of scattered caterpillars tend to attach themselves to larger ones, searching
aimlessly about for them, since they are unable to per-
ceive their fellow creatures beyond a certain distance.
If one caterpillar is kept in solitary captivity it builds a
nest alone, and appears to suffer no appreciable effect from
its isolation.   Among *Malocosoma* (Deegener, 1920) the caterpillars, even of different species, unite to form a " child
society ".   These insects often combine permanently with
companies of caterpillars belonging to another species.

   Young fishes not infrequently form " child families " ;
but families so created mingle with other members of their
own species the moment they meet, irrespective of whether
they are the offspring of the same or of different parents.

Herrings which have hatched out simultaneously remain permanently united, and thus form swarms differing from one another in the age of their members ; these swarms may mingle for a time, but each always re-issues intact from the mass. Young pythons keep together at first in a kind of community, later becoming solitary, like the parent snakes.

" Child families " are also found among mammals ; they might perhaps be more accurately designated " child herds " or herds of adolescents. Thus young cachalots sometimes live in groups of their own until sexually mature. Young roes stay with the mother until the next rutting season ; she then drives them away and they often unite to form herds of their own. Among wild reindeer the young males and females, not yet capable of reproduction, join together into herds of considerable size led by an old unmated female.

*a*3   *The Behaviour of Animals Debarred from Breeding*

Among many social mammals, but also among birds and reptiles (emerald lizards), old males are sometimes found living in solitude. Some authorities would consider mammals living thus as former leaders and harem-owners expelled by rebellious young males (Oedipus !). But since such solitary animals are found in so many different species it is probable that, in some cases, at least, weakening of the sexual impulse and a desire to abandon the restless life of the herd are important factors in their behaviour. In the mammalian species solitary animals are encountered among apes, elephants, buffaloes, deer, antelopes, giraffes, hippopotami, kangaroos, rodents, etc.

In the case of the gnu, males in their prime have been seen to expel older males from the herd and keep them away from it permanently (Schillings). The latter hold themselves aloof, like outposts, at a distance of a few hundred paces from the herd and give warning signals when danger approaches. Very old steers eventually separate themselves entirely from the herd and live a solitary life for the remainder of their days. Among bantin, the younger generation of bulls are said to make common cause against old steers and expel them from the herd.

Old males living unmated either keep strictly to themselves, or else seek out others in a like condition, whether the latter belong to their own or to another species. Old bull gnus, for instance, live in groups of twos and threes, and so do old bull elephants. Schilling saw two old bull elephants and an old male giraffe living together for weeks.

Among polygynous species there are always, in the nature of things, a large number of males which—for a time, at least, and possibly all their lives—are precluded from coition. Among sea-lions, and their allied species, where the male always collects a large harem, the excluded males gather together in two separate groups, one consisting of old, expelled, or wounded males, the other of the younger males, the " bachelors " as yet precluded from coition by the lords of the harems. Among guanacos the sexually mature young males expelled by the herd leader, foregather with others of their own age and with immature females. Young male vicunas remain with the mothers until they are full grown ; then, however, the whole herd of females unites to drive away the now sexually mature males with bites and kicks. These males then form herds of twenty or thirty head to which other unmated solitary males attach themselves after they have been defeated by a rival. These herds have no leader, and, at rutting time especially, live in a state of continuous quarrelling. Such " bachelor " herds are found among some species of apes, deer, antelopes, gazelles, and buffaloes. The troops of geldings found in South America, which herd together in companies of their own, and keep away from the harems, are, in a certain sense, " bachelor " herds. In Cape Colony adult male long-tailed monkeys are often met with living alone, and this has been taken to mean that they have been driven out of the herd by the " pachas ". Among migratory birds, those which, for some reason or another, have not paired, always return very early to their winter quarters.

Animals prevented from pairing and breeding often try, nevertheless, to satisfy their brooding instincts. Unmated guillemots are always to be found on the cliffs monopolized by this species for brooding, and they pounce upon any eggs temporarily abandoned by the parent birds, and brood for a little while. In Paraguay, female mules, though sterile, sometimes steal foals from mares ; they mother these foals, tender them their dry udders, etc., but the foals, of course, quickly perish. The German expression " ape-love ", connoting harmfully exaggerated parental care, does not, according to Brehm, refer to an ape mother's anxiety for her own offspring, but to the parental instinct which shows itself in childless apes ; these will appropriate the offspring of another female (sometimes belonging to a different species, or even the young of cats and dogs), thus gravely imperilling their lives, the would-be mothers having, for one thing, no milk to offer. Generally speaking, certain mammals, and also certain birds, show a striking tendency to adopt and tend anything young, more or less regardless of its size (Groos). The parental instinct is, therefore, awakened by whatever is young, awkward, or in need of help, and not by any special smallness of the animal. This instinct shows itself most clearly in individuals prevented, by some cause or another, from breeding.

2 The Behaviour of Seasonally Reproductive Species outside Breeding Time

The behaviour of seasonally reproductive species during the period of sexual inactivity varies greatly. Either the couples live in solitary monogamous mateships throughout the year and are abandoned by their children as soon as these have reached a certain stage of development (as in the case of some birds) ; or the family, consisting of father, mother, and children, remains united until the next pairing time in the following spring, possibly living gregariously, meanwhile, with other families. Alternatively the mates may separate after the breeding period and unite with others of their own sex to form male and female communities. Either the old mates reunite in the following season, or new mateships are formed from year to year. Whenever the females live in a herd of their own, accompanied by their young until the following spring or later, they form a " mother herd ".

a1 *Cases in which the Sexes Live Together*

Some fishes, living for a time in solitary mateships reunite after breeding time into large communities (e.g. the grayling, *Rhodeus amarus*). This is also true of some reptiles, e.g. lizards. Among sticklings and other species the males isolate themselves at breeding time, although outside this period they live a gregarious life.

Birds frequently assemble in flocks after the breeding season is over, sometimes only to fly from one haunt to another (in northern regions, titmice and some finches, in warmer latitudes, flamingoes), sometimes to migrate to more temperate zones. The migratory birds of the northern hemisphere naturally fly south in winter, those of the southern hemisphere north. Before they set out large crowds of them are seen to remain several days in the same spot. They migrate, according to the species, either in large masses of no particular shape, or in rows or in wedge formation ; in this last case the bird at the apex (whether male or female) is frequently relieved. Birds which have travelled together remain more or less united in their winter quarters. Migration is instinctive (C > V), for birds captured as nestlings and kept in isolation grow very restive as the migrating season approaches. It is not habit but instinct which determines the travel routes, at least among those species where every bird, including the young ones, sets out independently (see below).

With the settled warmth of spring, the birds break up their winter gatherings, whether these be formed for migrating or merely for feeding. The pairing of unmated birds is not a simple division of the winter flock into separate couples ; rather the gregarious impulse disappears and the mating impulse asserts itself more and more. Long-tailed tits (*Acredula caudata* and *rosea*) form societies during the winter which consist mainly of single families, i.e. parents with their young. In early spring these societies break up, and solitary unmated males are seen flying round alone in eager search for a mate, which, when found, they escort to the future nesting place (Haecker, p. 47). If, after their return in the spring, migratory birds are taken unawares by a recurrence of wintry weather, a number of couples living in the same area may be seen momentarily reunited in a common search for food (Haecker, p. 35).

In certain mammal species males and females unite to form societies between one pairing season and another Thus wolves, jackals, and hyenas live in hunting packs. I was able to see for myself, in the spring of 1915 after the Russian invasion of East Prussia, near Eydtkuhnen, that the instinct to form a hunting pack can be reawakened even in the domesticated dog. The district had been forsaken by its inhabitants, many farms had been burnt, and the cattle, and most of the dogs had perished. A few dogs, however, survived, and had formed themselves into packs of about a dozen which hunted over the fields like a line of infantry in open formation. It was a strange sight to see these packs composed as they were of dogs of all breeds, colours, and sizes, engaged in such a pursuit. Not one of these dogs had ever learned, either through tradition or upbringing, to hunt in this open formation ; but an ancient instinct prompted them, in their necessity, to form these hunting packs.

Among gregarious mammals the sexes very often separate after pairing time; nevertheless, among *Antilocapra americana* and saiga antelopes the two sexes are found living together throughout the year. The same thing occurs in the case of mammals living in colonies; the males and females do not separate. Many rodents, and also coneys (*Procavia*), live together in this way. Within such colonies the animals, alone (ground squirrels), or in couples (wild rabbits), dig a number of separate holes and burrows which are sometimes connected with one another, or several individuals may build a common dwelling. Dormice, alone or in companies, build ingenious nests in undergrowth; jerboas, and their allied species, wombats and opossums, live gregariously in holes which they dig themselves. Vizcachas and beavers live in colonies, the inhabitants of which are in close connexion with one another.

a2   Cases in which the Sexes Live Apart

The number of social species in which the sexes live apart, except at pairing time, is by no means small. It is, indeed not at all an infrequent occurrence for males on the one hand, and females on the other to form separate herds. If the females are accompanied by their young, a " mother herd " is the result. It is worth noting that societies composed of one sex only, and formed for no sexual purpose, are not restricted to man alone, but are also common among animals.

According to Schillings, for instance, among many antelopes the herds divide according to sex between one pairing time and another; it is true that a few bucks are occasionally found in the herds of females. Wild sheep, bouquetins, and other *Ungulata* likewise live, after the pairing season is over, in herds composed of one sex only. Among African and Indian elephants, too, the sexes form herds of their own, the herds of females being led by a female and accompanied by their young. In years past herds of several hundred head were often encountered, but they were the result of temporary alliances between several different troups.   In more recent times,   according to Schillings, the sorely decimated herds of East Africa probably no longer maintain the separation and classification of their societies according to age as strictly as in the days when they were more numerous.   If a herd of males and a herd of females chance to unite, the separation of the sexes is usually maintained, this being especially visible when the herd is resting.   Closer relations between the sexes occur only at breeding time, when a male temporarily takes possession of a herd of females to form his harem.

The bisons, which at one time were found by the million in North America, did not live in mere disorderly mobs. Every herd, however large, showed itself, on close inspection, to be composed of separate bands, each containing from six to sixteen bulls or thirty and more cows ; the bands of females were led by young males, and each band of males had also its own leader. In a large herd the troops of bulls formed an outer ring, whilst the cows herded together in the centre. Bison on the march, or grazing, generally moved in Indian file. It is said that at rutting time the herd did not divide into couples or harems ; nevertheless, the order described above must then have temporarily suffered considerable disorganization. Among seals, during the period of sexual inactivity, the sexes are encountered in separate herds. The females are accompanied by their young, and sometimes by the " bachelors ", i.e. males which did not succeed in mating. With Virginian deer the old males unite in herds of their own after rutting time, whereas the young males join the herds of females.

In some species the females live together with their young in " mother herds ", the younger, sexually mature males form herds of their own, and the older males live as hermits, seeking the herds of females only at pairing time. This is true of wild pigs, red deer, and fallow deer. Although bats are generally extremely social animals, after pairing time the male lives alone, and the females form swarms of their own in which no male has ever yet been found. Shortly before the outbreak of the great war, according to Brehm, in Bialowicza herds of female bison (*Bosbonasus*), an animal now extinct in its wild state, containing from ten to twenty head, were always led by an old cow and accompanied by two or three bulls. The younger bulls lived in herds numbering from fifteen to twenty, whereas the old bulls lived by themselves. Females were rarely encountered singly, and if they were it was probably as a result of the decimation of the species. At rutting time the old bulls joined the herds of females, and violent battles were fought for the possession of the latter. Other species of buffaloes are said to have the same habits. Among elks, in the winter, the males and the younger animals unite into herds, containing at the most fifty head, while the females often keep to themselves, each with its own offspring. Typical " mother herds " are found among some whales. Thus the cachalot appears in so-called "schools", numbering twenty or thirty animals, and entirely composed of females and their young; one old male acts as leader, called by whalers "the schoolmaster". Several schools may unite, each with its own schoolmaster. Schools of sperm whales have been seen, led by a female, and never accompanied by a male. In the case of the unsocial otter (*Lutra*), several females with their young often unite to form a " mother society " ; in the same way sportsmen occasionally encounter two or three lionesses and their young hunting together.

Some species of birds, when migrating, divide according to age and sex ; this habit has already been mentioned in connexion with chaffinches. In certain species old males on the one hand, and females and young males on the other, join together. It is common for the young birds to leave first, being followed a month or two later by the older birds, and last of all by the oldest males. In the spring this order is reversed. A typical instance of this is furnished by the starlings in Heligoland, whose period of migration extends from the end of June to December (Gaetke).

Wild turkey cocks unite after breeding time in societies of ten to a hundred, under the leadership of an old cock, while the hens collect in flocks with the half-grown young. In the course of the winter these groups, originally determined by sex, nevertheless mix with one another, but separate again before breeding time begins. Hand-reared cock pheasants, which are polygynous, abandon their mates and form flocks of males.

Some fishes live in shoals divided according to sex, e.g.

Leuciscus rutilus. When salmon come up from the sea, the sexes travel separately ; the shoals of males appear first, and are followed by the females ; it is said that they travel, like some birds, in V-formation.

a3   Societies composed of Different Species

We have seen that sometimes birds of different species brood together in the same colony. Other animal species, too, are found, especially at other than breeding time, living together, or with species whose rutting period is uninterrupted. We can here disregard those symbioses where the partners either exchange nourishment, or the one partner receives protection in exchange for foraging. We will only consider those cases where animals living their natural life unite mainly to satisfy their desire for companionship. We shall very soon discover that such societies may also possess biological significance. The links binding their members together are of varying strength, and consequently they must sometimes be classified rather as associations than as societies.

Different species of dolphins form troups led by one individual ; whales sometimes accompany ships, prompted by their " following instinct ". Antelopes of different species occasionally mix with one another ; the reed buck, which always keeps to itself, is an exception. The Peruvian prong-horned antelope joins herds of tame cattle, as does the elk. Wild zebras follow domesticated horses and graze among them. Gazelles mix with herds of cattle. Wild asses, different antelopes, yaks, and scattered horses

G

are sometimes seen together. Wild buffaloes associate with elephants.

Zebras live amicably with different species of gazelles, and with crested cranes ; these cases have sometimes been named " mutual assurance societies ", for the long-legged birds in question are guided by sight, the four-footed beasts by scent, and it may well be that what escapes the " eye " is detected by the " nose ". How far experience and tradition play a part in these societies is not known. Similarly antelopes and ostriches sometimes remain for hours in the midst of a troup of baboons (Schillings). Large flocks of *Ciconia abdimii* and white storks (*Ciconia alba*) often hunt grasshoppers together, as do white storks and marabouts. Stresemann has given a detailed account of the occurrence of bird flocks composed of different species.

In conclusion we may mention the herds of apes already described, which are composed of different species. Some apes, however, avoid those of other species, and two species of baboon, *hamadryas* and *gelada*, quarrel whenever they meet, shrieking and bellowing at each other, though they seldom actually come to blows.

VI SPECIAL ANIMAL SOCIOLOGY (*continued*)

B INSECT STATES

Insect states must be given a place apart in the sociology of animal species, for they are social structures of such complexity that they cannot be ranked with the animal societies already considered. Animal states exist only among insects; they possess, in consequence, certain common characteristics, however much they may differ in other respects. Thus they are always spatially circumscribed by the dimensions of the nest; further their members are always morphologically and psychologically highly differentiated, and are, in general, inconceivable apart from the community into which they are born. It is perhaps not inapt to regard insect states as families, or " super-families ". A bee-state would then be a mother family, and a termite state, in its simplest form, a parent family. But complications appear when, as among certain ants and termites, several egg-laying queens, or royal pairs, as the case may be, are present in the same community; or when insects of different origin unite to form one community, whether by reason of a slave raid, or in consequence of the adoption of a queen, or as a result of the peaceful fusion of two races. Any attempt at a rigid classification by relationship thus leads to great difficulties, and sometimes even to the separation of things in reality inseparable.

An insect community is divided into " estates " or castes, of which, in the simplest cases, there are three, males, females and workers. These estates or castes do not bear the smallest resemblance to those of human societies, for in these latter, to put it briefly, castes and estates continue to exist because they breed within themselves; thus the son is born into his father's caste. But in insect states the males and females form separate castes, and there is, in addition, a caste of workers, ordinarily sterile but reproducing themselves in certain special circumstances. Besides the workers some ants and termites have a special soldier class, also predominantly sterile. These two castes may fall into sub-castes, that is to say, into large, medium sized, and small workers and soldiers. It is characteristic of these insect castes that they do not breed within themselves, but that they all descend from the female. The term " caste " is, consequently, not very happily chosen.

These insect states are held together essentially not by tradition, but the extraordinary certainty of the instincts with which their members are endowed. The newly hatched individual knows from the outset all the essential things it must do or leave undone ; it never requires any kind of tuition (C, therefore, largely outweighs V). It is this above all which is so puzzling in the study of insect life.

Our chief problem, in this connexion, is as follows : how is it that, in insect states, the activities of every insect are almost invariably directed towards a common end ? Who, at the proper moment, gives the word of command ? An actual leader is lacking ; to call the female " the queen " is totally misleading, she is usually no more than an egg-

laying machine, at least when the size of the community
increases. Among white ants the " king " has no other
function than that of fecundating the female from time to
time. We are driven, then, to the following supposition ;
in spite of some individual differences in temperament
and native endowment, the members of an insect community
are, in general, psychically so closely attuned to one another
that when one insect gives a particular signal this is sufficient
at once to induce in all the rest a like series of movements.
Likewise when the same external stimulus affects them,
they all behave either similarly, or in a manner dictated
by a common purpose. That which prompts this organized
activity is, therefore, neither a command nor an intellectual
operation, but a common store of instincts which every
individual possesses, and their mutual adaptation to one
another, which we might call an interlocking of instincts.

1 Rudimentary States : Humble Bees

The majority of wasps and bees are solitary ; only a few
are social. In the solitary species relations between
individuals occur only when male and female come together
in the act of coition. Mother and children, as a rule,
know nothing of one another. It is true that some solitary
bees show a rudimentary form of social life, since they
nest in colonies and make common cause against aggressors,
and also sleep and hibernate together. Some solitary
wasps hunt in common, although this does not prevent them
from robbing one another on the return journey. (For
other rudimentary types of society see von Buttel-Reepen,
Friese, Peckham, and Wheeler.)

The humble bee state lasts only a year.   The fecundated young female (the queen) winters alone, and in the spring builds a nest by herself.   She maintains relations with her offspring by subsequently reopening the previously sealed waxen cells in which the eggs were laid, and feeding the young.   This nourishment is, however, insufficient, and the young emerge as small female workers, only able to reproduce themselves by parthenogenesis.   Thenceforward they do all the work, and thus play the same part as that of the workers in communities of bees, ants and termites.   The queen thenceforward confines herself to laying eggs.   There is a division of labour among the female workers : some only look after the larvæ, others build, and others again fly abroad, collecting food ;   sometimes honey is brought in and stored.   Workers whose nest has been destroyed will take shelter in other nests, possibly even in those of a different species.   Later in the year, as a result of better feeding, large females, capable of reproduction, and males, are hatched out, the latter from the unfertilized eggs of the queen and the workers.   Coition takes place in the open air.   In the autumn the whole community perishes with the exception of the young fecundated females.

A great deal of discussion centred at one time round the so-called " trumpeter " of humble bees.   Early every morning a bee appears at the entrance of the nest and there produces a loud humming by the rapid beating of its wings.   This does not, as was once imagined, serve the purpose of a reveillé ; the insect merely acts as a living ventilator, and if it is captured another takes its place.

2 Bees

The honey bee state may be described, at a certain stage at least, as a mother family (v. Buttel-Reepen, Jordan, Doflein, Deegener). At first the queen is surrounded by her sisters (the sterile worker bees) alone. These are later joined by her own children (males, females and workers), and at the end of the season her children only (i.e. workers) people the hive. Among honey bees the queen is never left alone, but is always surrounded by a swarm of workers, which guard, clean and feed her ; she devotes herself solely to propagation. A well-stocked hive contains from 20–75,000 workers ; they alone are equipped for foraging, and are degenerated and sterile females.

These workers build the cells for storing food and the cells for the offspring ; the queen lays an unfertilized egg in each drone cell, and a fertilized egg in each worker and in each queen cell. She can either fertilize the egg as it emerges by semen contained in a special sac, or leave it unfertilized. For six or eight weeks she lays about two thousand eggs a day, and this daily output weighs twice as much as her own body.

The care of the brood and the entire economy of the hive falls to the lot of the workers. A special instinct for cleanliness prompts them to keep the hive clean, and besides this they clean themselves and each other. The young bees busy themselves within the hive, while the older ones (the foragers) fly abroad. Of the food brought into the hive, part is converted into an artificial food, part is consumed by the foragers themselves, and part is given to the other workers. Bee-bread and honey are produced in this way. Honey is manufactured from nectar, and is prepared in the proventriculus, or crop, of the workers. The thickening of the honey takes place not only in the crop, but also in the cells to which it is brought, and which remain open for a time before being sealed ; the necessary air supply is provided by a number of workers rhythmically beating their wings. Honey is produced both for current consumption and for storing in reserve. Bee-bread is made of pollen which some of the bees bring in and deposit in the cells, while others, whose activities are confined to the hive, pack it tight and seal it over. The foraging bees occasionally penetrate into neighbouring hives and steal honey. Bee hives with only a small population may suffer severely from such marauders.

The unfertilized eggs produce drones, the fertilized eggs females or workers. Whether a female or a worker is to be reared from the fertilized egg depends in the first instance upon lodging it in an appropriate cell, and then upon the kind of nourishment supplied to the larva. Each of the three different types of larva is provided with an appropriate diet by the bees tending the brood. Every young worker larva can be developed into a queen by the worker bees ; they have only to transform its cell into a " queen-cell " and provide it with the food supplied to the queens. Like the larvæ, both the drones and the queens have to be fed by the worker bees, which supply them with chyle (bee-bread partially digested in the second stomach and regurgitated) ; the chyle is also used in feeding the young.

Every year from two to six queens are reared in succession As soon as one is full grown she emits a piping sound in her cell, and this throws the whole community into a state of the greatest excitement. The old queen always attempts to kill the young one, but the latter is protected by a guard of workers ; she then forsakes the hive, accompanied by ten or fifteen thousand bees. This swarm attaches itself in a grape-like cluster to a branch, or some similar object, and subsequently settles in a new home which has been explored two or three days beforehand by a few bees acting as scouts or forerunners (unless, of course, the bee-keeper houses it by force in a new hive). The young queen left in the hive attacks the remaining queen cells and kills the females developing within them. The workers prevent this only if the hive is sufficiently populous to allow of the formation of a second swarm ; in this case the next queen to appear departs with a second swarm, and her successor sometimes again with a third. The queen finally left in possession of the hive never fails to destroy every female still in course of development. In any one bee state there is but one queen.

If the queen does not fly out with the swarm the bees return to the mother hive ; this also happens if the queen perishes before any young larvæ have come into existence. If more than one queen (the old one and several young ones) flies out with the swarm, all but one are killed. Should the queen be removed, or die, the greatest excitement takes possession of the hive. Each individual emits a peculiar and characteristic sound (the mourning cry) so that the loss is immediately known all over the hive. If a substitute queen is introduced she is at first treated with enmity, but after a day, or a day and a half, she is accepted. If, on the death of a queen, the hive remains queenless too long, many of the workers lay unfertilized eggs, and any new queen is rejected ; the stock then quickly perishes. Among stingless bees, the *Meliponæ*, the old queen does not depart with the swarm ; it is the young queens that fly off, surrounded by part of the community.

Among honey bees the new queen is fecundated during the nuptial flight by a drone in a single copulation, after which she returns to the hive. The remaining drones are subsequently destroyed by the workers. The massacre of the drones does not usually take the form of stinging them to death, rather they are driven by the workers out of the hive into the open air, and there they perish.

The smell of the nest serves as a mark of identification among bees belonging to the same hive. It is a blend of the smell of each individual and that of the nest in general (including that of the brood, the wax and the food). All strange bees which lack this particular smell are slain, for sentinels, stationed at the entrance of the hive (as happens among all other social insects), examine every arrival unless the numbers in the hive have too greatly weakened. If the bee-master wishes to provide a new queen for a queenless hive, he must first place her in the hive for a day or two, confined in a small wire cage, so that she may acquire the smell of the nest or that a mutual exchange of smell may take place ; otherwise she will be put to death.

3 Ants

Among ants several queens are sometimes found in the same state (Escherich, Forel, Wasmann, Wheeler, Doflein, and others). These may have come from different nests,

having combined together after fecundation. Sexually
mature males remain in the community for a short time only.
as they leave the nest for ever after a few days, pair, and die.
The number of workers which a nest may contain varies
from a few dozen to several hundred thousand ; if the
inhabitants of daughter colonies living in amity with those
of the mother nest are included in the reckoning, the whole
population frequently numbers several, or even many (up
to one hundred) millions.

The workers, as with bees, are specially adapted, sterile
females ; they are, however, wingless, unlike the normal
males and females. A far-reaching division of labour is the
rule among the workers ; their apportioned tasks are either
feeding and cleaning the larvæ, building, or foraging. The
younger ones are first kept occupied within the nest, and only
the elder ones are sent abroad. The males seldom perform
any social duty, though they do, for example, help in carrying
the young in changing from one nest to another ; the females,
on the other hand, often assist in the work of the community ;
they help in building, and in times of danger carry larvæ
and chrysalides. The division of labour is, in some species,
connected with a morphological polymorphism in the
workers ; two, three, or more types are then found. Thus
in the case of *Atta*, the middle-sized workers are leaf-cutters,
the large ones leaf-grinders, and the smallest tend the
fungus-gardens. Soldiers, again, are a special type.

The excitement of the males and females preparing for the
nuptial flight spreads to the workers ; during this time
practically no work is done. The males and females do not
depart all at once, but gradually. The inhabitants of

different nests collect in great swarms in the air. There, during the nuptial flight, enmities based upon a difference of nest smell cease to exist. The queen may be fecundated by more than one male. After her fecundation she throws off her wings and proceeds to found a new colony, sometimes combining with other females for this purpose. She lays eggs, and nourishes herself and the first born larvæ upon some of the eggs she has herself produced ; afterwards the rising generation of workers undertakes each its appointed task. When several queens found a colony together they live peaceably with one another until the first workers begin to appear ; after that, however, they commonly fight until all but one are killed. Should it happen that one colony contains several queens at a time when outward circumstances are unfavourable, all but one are slain by the workers.

There are certain species in which the female is incapable of rearing its own brood ; such a " dependent " queen takes refuge with a female of another species still possessing the power to do so, and leaves her brood to be reared by the latter. In extreme cases the workers, too, of the given species have lost the instinct to tend the young, and the work devolves entirely upon the workers of the second species. Alternatively a " dependent " queen has to permit herself to be adopted by workers who have lost their own queen, and with their help found her new colony ; or again she may steal a few chrysalides of another species, and rear them into worker ants for her own service. Sometimes a queen will enter a nest, kill all its full-grown inhabitants, and rear the larvæ into workers to serve her. Under certain conditions the workers also lay eggs. Very many eggs are eaten by the ants themselves ; an ant will even eat the egg it has just laid.

The workers keep the nest scrupulously clean ; they feed and cleanse the young, and move them, several times a day, from one chamber into another of a more appropriate temperature or humidity ; the brood is housed according to age and size, in chambers which provide the environment most suitable to each stage of their development. The workers help the larvæ to spin their cocoons, and assist the full-grown insects to emerge from the chrysalis. In monogynous communities the death of the queen directly affects the welfare of the workers ; their ordered activities cease forthwith, and soon afterwards they die.

The building instinct among ants is highly adaptable ; the nests are, in consequence, particularly well suited to their surroundings. The foundation of a colony may take place as the result of the division of an existing state ; as many as sixteen hundred nests have been counted, all connected with one another, and possessing between them a population of many millions. It may happen that the friendliest relations between the inmates of one branch nest and another may change, in time, to enmity. In the course of a foray, ants of one species will take forcible possession of a nest belonging to another species. Every change of nest involves a procession of all the inhabitants carrying with them eggs, larvæ, and chrysalides

Weaver ants belong to the rare class of tool-using animals, and the tool they use is one of their own larvæ. They weave together leaves, each of a number of workers seizing a larva and using it in the process, whilst other workers hold the edges of the leaves together. If the space between the leaves is greater than the body of the ant, as many as eight form a chain, each clasping its neighbour's waist with its jaws.

Individuals belonging to different nests, even when they belong to the same species, usually dislike one another; boundary disputes and thefts of stores frequently occur, the latter either during transport, or even from the nest itself; a war may be carried on between two nests for months; if neither side is vanquished, mutual toleration, or even friendship may ensue. Alliances between two different states are, indeed, not exceptional.

Some species hunt singly, others in swarms, e.g. the wandering ants; in the last case even rats and mice can be overpowered, and the flesh carried off in small fragments. Ants belonging to the same nest feed one another, the food being passed from mouth to mouth. Forel is, therefore, not altogether unjustified in describing the crop as a " social stomach ", since one insect does feed another from it; only food reaching the digestive stomach benefits the individual itself, and Forel consequently called this portion of the alimentary canal the " private stomach ". A hungry ant " begs " from a full fed comrade by striking it sharply on the surface of the body and the side of the head with its forelegs and antennæ and licking its mouth, whereupon the other promptly feeds it. A full fed ant will pass on part of its stores to others, and repeat the process several times. Those species which invariably employ slaves to do the work of the state are absolutely dependent upon the latter for food. The brood-tending ants feed the larvæ by vomiting a drop of fluid and letting it fall into their mouths. In

species where the lárvæ possess solid jaws they are also
fed with dead insects and the like. It is not yet known
whether the workers develop females, and the various types
of worker and soldier grubs, by varying the fluid on which
these are fed.

Ants make provision for the future purely instinctively ;
they are " breeders " in the sense that they rear and tend
insects whose excretions are sweet to the taste. They lay
up stores of seed and honey, and cultivate fungi ; and they
help each other to carry home prey.

An ant " milking " an aphide, i.e. inducing it to excrete,
taps the hinder portion of the aphide's body with its
antennæ ; the aphis then lifts its hind parts and evácuates
from its anus a yellowish drop of excrement, which is always
rich in sugar. The ants protect and guard the aphides, and
if necessary bring them into safety ; they build strong
defences round them, carry their eggs into the nest in winter,
and in the spring deposit the young aphides on plants.
Young, newly hatched ants, without previous instruction,
treat aphides' eggs in exactly the same way that the older
experienced workers do, so that here there is no question
of imitation. Root-eating aphides are kept by ants in suitable
places within the nest itself. Some species of ants live entirely
upon aphis excrement, and there are, correspondingly, some
species of leaf- and root-eating aphides which cannot exist
apart from their association with ants. Ants also devour
the sweet excrement of some cicadas ; one species of ant
builds special nests of leaves for the rearing of these insects.
Some ants also feed upon the glandular secretions of the
caterpillars of certain butterflies. The caterpillars are

guarded by the ants in question, and are dragged into the nest before the chrysalis stage in order that they may complete their metamorphosis undisturbed.

Honey ants (*Myrmecocystus*), found in Colorado, gather the sweet liquid which is exuded by the gall formed by *Cyrips tinctaria* on dwarf oaks.   Any portion not immediately consumed is stored in the crops of special workers, the "honey-carriers". These, in the beginning normal young workers, are fed until their crops are so full that the whole of the hinder part of the body is swollen completely out of shape, and in this condition they hang for the greater part of their lives, immobile, from the ceilings of special store rooms. Should external supplies of food fail, the population lives upon the contents of the crops of the honey-carriers, allowing themselves to be fed by the latter.

The grain collecting species, which are found in warm countries, either seek together in the open air for seeds, or raid the granaries of other ant states and of men. The grain brought into the nest is cleaned and shelled by a special subordinate caste of workers ; it is prevented from germinating by the dryness of the chambers used by the ants as granaries. The ants probably cause it to germinate by moistening it before they consume it.

Leaf-cutting ants are agriculturists in the sense that they cultivate a kind of fungus. The fungus gardens are situated within their nests, and the workers sow and tend a particular kind of fungus which they grow upon specially prepared soil. This fungus occurs only in ants' nests, and for this reason a queen, setting forth to found a new nest, must take with her a piece of the plant ; this she carries in a pouch in her mouth. The soil in question is prepared from fragments of leaves which the workers cut in the open air and then knead into soft lumps. This soil has to be frequently renewed and " weeded " to keep it free from other fungi and bacteria. The division of labour between the large, medium-sized, and small *Atta* workers has already been described. The *Atta* ants feed solely upon small tumours which appear on the fungi (the so-called " turnips "), which are very rich in albumen. Other species of ants besides *Atta* cultivate fungi, preparing the necessary soil from powdered wood and the excrement of wood-eating insects.

The worker ants clean and lick themselves and each other freely, and bestow a similar care upon the queen and the brood ; this licking, however, cannot be attributed solely to a desire for cleanliness, but rather to the presence of certain skin secretions which induce this action. Refuse is taken out of the nest or brought to remote places within it and there sometimes covered with earth ; dead ants are treated in the same way. These habits are the substantial element in certain highly imaginative descriptions of ant funerals and ant cemeteries.

If the nest is invaded the brood and the females are placed in safety in the deepest recesses of the nest, or else the inmates try to escape, taking the brood and the females with them. If the nest is inundated, the ants form themselves into living balls, with the brood and the females well protected in the centre. They broadcast an alarm throughout the nest by tapping one another with their antennæ, or by making knocking noises, or by using a special chirping organ with which they are equipped. The inhabitants of a nest differ considerably from one another in temperament and courage ; the latter quality, as among all social animals, grows in proportion to the number of comrades fighting together.   Their battle fury may rise to a veritable intoxication ; when this stage is reached, the ants throw themselves upon their infuriated companions, and hold them fast until the madness passes. An ant which has lost its way in the open is carried back to the nest by a companion.   A sort of nursing of the sick unmistakably occurs among ants, any that are ill or damaged being tended and licked. Care of this kind seems, however, actually to be limited to cases which are not desperate, for the badly wounded, and some of the sick, are left unattended, or are carried off, without a moment's delay, to the rubbish heap. Ants, as I have said in the introduction, do not remove mites, or other harmful parasites from one another's bodies. Those most familiar with the habits of ants assert unhesitatingly that they play together.   Judgments of this kind cannot be too circumspect, but the mock battles which take place among the inhabitants of one nest during warm weather, and when they are undisturbed, seem to be quite justifiably described as play.

A mixed colony arises when the workers of one colony receive into their midst a female belonging to another (adoption of a queen) ; it may also arise out of an alliance, or out of a conquest.   The larvæ stolen on a well-organized "slave raid" are some of them reared, and some of them eaten.   The so-called slaves are fully franchised "citizens" of the ant states in which they have shed their cocoons, and are not slaves in the sense in which the word is understood when applied to human societies. The presence of these slaves in an ant state is not comparable with the employment of natives as soldiers and officials by civilized occidentals, for natives are always regarded, though in varying degrees, as citizens of an inferior order.

The genus *Polyergus* is an " obligatory slave-keeper ", since the workers are only capable of stealing larvæ and cocoons, and depend entirely on their slaves for food ; without them they would die of starvation. The genus *Anergates* has only males and females, no workers. A female of this species penetrates into a *Tetramorium* colony, and is adopted by its workers, who probably even kill their former queen. A female *Anergates* produces only males and females, which have all to be fed by the *Tetramorium* workers. Gradually the *Tetramorium* colony dies out for lack of progeny, and the *Anergates* males and females in its midst are doomed along with their hosts. One or other of the *Tetramorium* females alone escapes death by migrating to another *Tetramorium* colony.

There are numerous insect species, the *Myrmekophila* (Wasmann), which live with ants. The individuals of these species are never found living together alone, but always associated with ants. These guests of the ant are sometimes so dependent upon this mode of life that they are incapable of existing apart from their hosts. Myrmecophilous insects can be divided into three classes. (1) Synecthrans, which are directly harmful to their hosts, and which these latter encounter with hostility. (2) Synoekites, whose presence either does not affect the ants in any way, or at least is neither specially harmful nor specially useful to them ;

these are tolerated by their hosts. (3) Symphiles, or true guests of the ant. All symphilous insects exude aromatic volatile substances ; these exudations take place from special hairs, the *trichomæ*, which grow in stiff bunches. For the sake of these exudations the ants do not merely tolerate the existence of symphilous insects, but even look after them, and in time of danger rescue them with the brood. As the exudations are brought forth only in very small quantities they are not a necessity but a luxury ; the craving for them may amount to a social evil in an ant state, and for this reason Escherich compares it with the passion for alcohol and opium among men ; it sometimes costs the ant state not only a part of its nourishment, but also its brood. Symphilous instincts among ants must be regarded as differentiations of the general brood-tending and adopting instincts.

Wasmann takes the relation between the beetle *Lomechusa strumosa*, and the ant *Formica sanguinea*, as a classic example of symphilia. The ants feed the beetles from their crops and tend their young with greater zeal than they do their own brood, even though the *Lomechusa* larvæ devour the eggs and larvæ of the ants in large quantities. This aberration of the normal brood-tending instinct results eventually in the production of a stunted type of ant intermediate between a worker and a female, the pseudogynæ. In this way the ant colony eventually perishes from degeneration, and the *Lomechusa* migrate to another nest. Some of these parasites, e.g. the beetles *Lomechusa* and *Clavigera*, adapt themselves so completely to the habits of their hosts that they make use of their antennæ to tap the ants with which they come into contact just as these do each other.

As I have already said, ants belonging to different nests, even when members of the same species, are hostile to one another ; they rob one another of aphides and stores and brood, and go so far as to drive one another out of their nests. Before an organized foray, scouts spy out a favourable moment for the attack. Inhabitants of the same nest recognize one another by the special nest odour, which, as among bees, is a compound of that of the individual and that of the nest. Sentinels stand at the entrance of the ant-hill and drive away all who do not bear the " uniform " of the special nest odour. Ants which have been kept isolated from their nest comrades are welcomed by the latter months or years later. Where this does not happen it is to be supposed that the returned wanderer has lost the nest odour in the interval. In a mixed colony there is a special mixed smell, and on this account masters and slaves of different species live peacefully together in the same state, provided they all possess an identical "livery of smell " ; they will make common cause against the inmates of another state, even though they belong to different species.

It is possible to create artificially mixed colonies by placing together young ants, only just out of the cocoon, in an artificial nest, for they do not then possess any special nest odour ; either they have not as yet acquired it, or it may not yet have been formed. Mixed colonies of older ants can be created by thoroughly shaking representatives of different species together in a sack, whereby the different nest odours blend with one another ; but it is true that this experiment does not succeed with all species. It has never been found possible to create mixed colonies of ants and termites.

Ants do not always allow their behaviour towards other ants to be guided blindly by the nest odour. If a few individuals of different species are put together into an enclosed space their desire for companionship often conquers their mutual hostility. Should a female, incapable of founding a colony by herself, enter the nest of another species which has lost its queen, she is not put to death, but adopted. Peace may be spontaneously concluded between two nests which have carried on a long and indecisive war, or between two nests simultaneously menaced by a common enemy. In such a contingency the hitherto hostile tribe is recognized by its smell and duly respected. The means of mutual understanding which ants possess in the shape of their " antennæ language " will be dealt with in a special section of my General Animal Sociology.

4 Termites

Termites (Escherich, Doflein, Deegener) provide an interesting parallel to ants, and for this reason they have been called " white ants ", although the two species have strictly no connexion with one another. Some of the resemblances between them are very striking, and provide us with what is, perhaps, our most impressive instance of convergent evolution between two animal groups, the similarity of whose habits has produced similar morphological and biological characteristics. Unfortunately we are still very ignorant of the psychology of termites, which is especially regrettable for present purposes.

A single termite state may contain only a few hundreds of inhabitants, but in the case of tropical species these may number millions or even milliards. In addition to winged males and females there are sterile and wingless workers and soldiers which are specially modified males and females, divided, sometimes, into sub-castes. The workers are able to produce recruits for all the various castes from the sexless young; and they are even capable of rearing substitute males and females from worker and soldier larvæ, and soldiers from male and female larvæ, probably by varying the nourishment with which they supply them. The workers are careful to maintain the proper numerical proportion between the number of individuals in each caste ; if there are too many in any one caste the superfluous insects are killed and eaten ; if there are too few the scarcity is relieved by the transmutation already described.

The functions of the workers are nest-building, gathering food, cleaning and feeding the males, females and soldiers, tending the brood and keeping the hive clean. The larger workers busy themselves outside, and the small workers inside, the nest ; the latter is defended by the soldiers, which are incapable of feeding themselves. The soldiers are sub-divided into classes according to size ; the outer defences are manned by the larger types, whereas the medium-sized and smaller ones police the interior of the nest ; these latter supervise the groups of workers, urging on idlers with taps of their antennæ. Under the supervision of the smaller soldiers, workers take in charge the eggs laid by the queen ; larger soldiers surround the king and queen, and defend them if necessary. The sentinels posted at the entrance give the alarm when danger approaches by tapping and chirping.

After swarming both male and female shed their wings, remain together as a pair, and often only attain sexual maturity after a period which may extend from a fortnight to five months. The pair hide themselves and dig themselves in together. When the first eggs hatch out, brooding instincts appear in both males and females ; later the adult workers assume responsibility for the offspring. From one to six pairs have been found in the same nest. In many species the queen lays an egg every two seconds, and may continue doing so for years. Every pair copulates repeatedly, and lives monogamously unless one of the partners dies. If the queen perishes the king is provided with a number of substitute queens (as many as a hundred) and lives henceforward polygynously. If both king and queen die, numerous substitute pairs arise in their stead.

In cases of necessity, i.e. when the king or the queen, or both, die, substitute males and females are generally reared from a special type of larvæ held in reserve. Worker or soldier larvæ are seldom converted into substitute males or females. Sometimes a winged male or female couple is prevented from leaving the nest to swarm and is put by force in the place of a pair which have died. In some species a " substitute " type exists side by side with the normal males and females, whereas in other species no such type is ever found. Soldiers also, on occasion, lay eggs.

Colonies are sometimes founded by a secession from the mother nest ; in this case a number of workers, taking with them eggs and larvæ, form a new nest, which is at first closely connected with the old one, but later becomes totally independent. A new royal couple is created for the new nest from substitute males and females; sometimes a young pair is adopted from outside.

Termite workers devour their sickly and dead companions. They feed the larvæ, the males and females, the soldiers, and their fellow workers by regurgitation or, in the case of wood-eating species, by defecation. In these species the excrement always contains a considerable amount of nutriment. One ant " begs " excrement of another by stroking the hinder part of its companion's body with antennæ and feelers. The flow of excrement may be produced experimentally with the help of a paint brush. Excrement and vomit are also used in nest-building.

Termites, like ants, construct store-chambers. With termites these contain fragments of finely shredded grass and leaves or grain and other seeds. Termites also cultivate fungi; the soil they use is vegetable matter reduced to very small pieces. These fungus gardens must be diligently weeded, for if they are removed from the care of the termites they run wild in a very short time. It would appear that, besides weeding, some complicated process of cultivation is needed; for the small knots which appear on the fungi and are used as food for the queen and the young brood, grow only under the care of the termites.

Individual termites belonging to the same nest also know one another by a special nest odour; strangers which do not possess this smell are killed. Ants and termites are one another's greatest enemies, ants always being the aggressors. Termitophila are found associated with termites. As among ants, three different species can be distinguished : (1) the synecthrans, (2) the synoekites, and (3) the symphiles. The last exude secretions. The growth of special hairs is more or less absent among the real guests of the termites ; exudation takes place through pores in the skin, but here, too, in such small quantities as only to provide a luxury, not a necessity. The termites nourish the symphiles on royal food, tend them, lick them, and sometimes rear them. These are harmful chiefly because they often attack the termite brood. Symphiles are nearly always beetles of one kind or another, but may also be flies, or a species of butterfly. Among termites as among ants, certain insects are used as " milch cows " ; the termites visit these insects outside the nest, or keep them inside it for the sake of their excreta.

VII GENERAL ANIMAL SOCIOLOGY

In this section I shall give an account of the general features which characterize the social life of animals. This science is still, unfortunately, in its infancy, and consequently what we have here to offer cannot be compared with the very substantial achievements of human sociology. Yet we can even now state various facts of very great interest from the point of view of comparative group psychology.

A THE SOCIETY OR THE COMMUNITY

A distinction has been drawn above between associations and societies; the first are chance aggregations in the sense that they are brought together by external environmental factors (light, warmth, nourishment, etc.), whereas societies hold together because all their members possess special social instincts. Societies may be classified as (1) closed or (2) open communities. In the first case it is only under special conditions that new members are admitted, or that a member, once incorporated, withdraws; furthermore a well-defined hierarchy is very often found to exist. In an open society, on the contrary, the members come and go without any special difficulties; it is therefore possible to distinguish between (a) organized and (b) unorganized communities; in the first the individuals have each their appointed status, in the second there is no such arrangement. Considering the difficulty of making clear-cut lines of

107

demarcation in the natural world, this division is, I think, not excessively artificial.

The community is held together, and its members are able to recognize one another chiefly by means of either the sense of smell (insects, many gregarious mammals) or the sense of sight (especially among birds). The sense of hearing often forms a useful auxiliary, and the more or less perfect development of the sense is coincident, among many social animals, with the possession of characteristic vocal organs. The horse whinnies if separated from his stable companion, and thus gives expression to the frustration of his social instincts ; a dog unaccustomed to loneliness, howls ; birds sound notes of invitation or warning as occasion requires ; a goat, alone in a stable, moans, but give it a rabbit for company and it is soothed at once. The goat and the rabbit do not enter into any closer relation ; the fact that another living creature is present is sufficient to allay the goat's desire for companionship. In Java macaques are often kept in stables ; the Javanese say that this prevents the horses from becoming bored, and makes them thrive better.

Whether or not individuals of the same species recognize one another as members of the same community in many cases does not seem to depend upon their colouring ; otherwise it would be impossible for albinos to appear, as they occasionally do, in flocks of birds (among sparrows, cranes, etc.). Moreover, under natural conditions, the males of the species *Machetes pugnax* are quite differently coloured and yet associate freely with one another. Domesticated fowls, ducks and pigeons recognize their comrades in spite of differences of colouring, and this is also true of domesticated dogs. The homogeneity of a species, in spite of the varied appearance of its members to human vision, is conditioned by their whole demeanour, and among dogs, also by a similarity of odour. I have to thank Dr. Drost, of Heligoland, for the following communications bearing upon this point. During marking experiments carried out upon migratory birds taken from the bird sanctuary there, a number of the birds are painted different colours in order to make them specially recognizable. These birds are always admitted by others of the same species to the communities to which they belong (e.g. peewits painted red). The same holds good for domesticated fowls which had been painted in order to carry out preliminary experiments. Thus if birds cease to be recognized by their own kind it must be for other reasons than that of a mere difference in colouring (for further details see below).

1 Closed Societies

The closed society is a community shut against non-members. These are either totally excluded, or gain admittance only with great difficulty. Within such a community there is often an established hierarchy ; among birds it is likely that this is always the case, but it probably never occurs among insects.

Insect states are closed societies. As we saw in the section which dealt with them, inmates of the same nest or hive recognize one another by a separate and distinct nest odour, even when the state to which they belong contains millions of inhabitants, for inmates of the same nest bear the same " uniform of smell ". Mutual tolerance, therefore, does not depend upon recognition of one another by the individuals concerned. Membership of the same community, and not membership of the same species, decides whether two animals shall tolerate or shall fight each other ; this is particularly clear in the mixed colonies of ants, where different species may be citizens of one and the same state, and hold together through thick and thin.

Single bees, isolated from the hive, soon die. They live longer if they have access to the odour of the hive and to that of the queen in particular. It is quite unnecessary that they should be near the hive and the queen, the odour has merely to attach to their prison. Solitary bees, on the contrary, bear isolation without any ill-effect.

According to Goetsch, mere solitude does not shorten the life of ants if they are given earth and brood with which to satisfy their building and brood-tending instincts.   If either of these instincts remains unappeased they die. They perish more quickly when both building material and brood are lacking.   Ants will remain alive under the most un-favourable conditions if, in addition to building materials, they are given a queen and brood. Where a queen and brood are lacking the cause of death is perhaps the want of those substances which the ants lick from their bodies rather than the impossibility of satisfying their tending instincts.   If a new queen is placed in a nest which has been long without one, the workers cannot lick her enough.

Solitary monogamous mateships and families, and solitary harems are closed societies.   In these the parents always know their own young ; some parents, e.g. ostriches, bite and kill young which do not belong to them. Hordes which inhabit a special area and defend it against intruders are closed societies. We may include here those animal communities whose members have been thrown together by chance within the same cage, and have there formed an organized society. Mutual recognition and tolerance in all such cases is the result of the individuals knowing each other.

The half-wild pariah dogs of the East, according to Brehm, immediately attack any of their kind which have not grown up with them, and which, so to speak, have not scuffled together with them. Thus in oriental cities every street and alley has its own pack of half-wild dogs, which never leave it. If one of these dogs enters a strange alley, the dogs domiciled there fall upon the stranger and tear it to pieces unless it saves itself by speedy flight. Penguins behave in just the same way during their breeding time. They brood, as earlier described, in gigantic colonies which are traversed by numerous pathways cutting each other at right-angles. Each of the resulting rectangles is the home of a pair of penguins. The birds in the neighbouring rectangles are manifestly more closely connected with one another than with the rest of the birds in the brooding colony ; but if a penguin strays into a more distant block of nests where it has no right of abode, it is fiercely expelled.

A society often has a leader. We saw that among mammals this may be either a male or a female, according to the species. Often the strongest and most experienced animal holds this rank. But from certain observations made by Schjelderup-Ebbe on fowls, to be discussed later, we may infer that strength and experience are not the only qualification necessary, but that in addition a specific aptitude for leadership is involved. Among fowls, physical strength alone does not determine the status of an individual in the " pecking order " ; psychic factors are more important. In those hordes of apes which are composed of several harems, each with its own pacha, the latter rules only his own family. Each harem is more closely united within itself than with the remaining harems, and yet the old males together watch over and fight for the safety of the whole horde. Among Arabian baboons, when a horde is on the march, a few old males lead the way, others remain in the rear, while others again are posted as sentinels at elevated spots. In case of danger every full-grown male makes for the threatened point. When the horde takes to flight the old apes deal out cuffs and blows to the younger and less experienced, forcing them thereby to hasten their movements (Schillings). Wounded and dead companions are borne along with the horde, and this does not apply only to mothers and their young. According to Brehm, an old male Arabian baboon which had been wounded supported himself right and left upon young apes, and boxed their ears whenever any detail of the flight was not carried out according to his wishes.

If an animal seeks admittance to an already established closed society it is, as a rule, initially received with great hostility. Schulz added a third to two young rhinoceroses who were used to one another ; these two immediately attacked the new arrival and harmony and friendship were not established until later. The same thing happens if a new animal is placed in the common cage of a zoological garden.

Apes and beasts of prey, also prairie marmots, parrots, etc., hurl themselves immediately upon any new-comer of their own species or breed, and ill-treat it or bite it to death. If the stranger survives this reception, peace is often established only after a great deal of scuffling ; possibly such battles are always waged with a view to establishing degrees of superiority (see below Schjelderup-Ebbe on hens and ducks) ; according to Pfungst every ape " knows its place " within the herd.

According to Köhler, a chimpanzee kept in solitary confinement is no true chimpanzee and becomes such only as a member of a group. The same is true, in greater or lesser degree, of all social animals, and of men. The actions of other members of its own species are, for every individual, the sole stimuli capable of prompting a large number of vital activities ; group solidarity is a real force of the greatest importance.

The chimpanzees kept in the experimental station at Teneriffe when first procured were quite young ; they might be called children (Rothmann and Teuber, Köhler). In the early days of their captivity they tended to form a herd, but this tendency disappeared as they became more familiar with one another, and an elder male took the lead. Once they had trodden out paths on their allotted patch of grass, they stuck to them. It was noteworthy that each of the animals possessed a strongly marked individuality. The group, therefore, was in no sense homogeneous ; rather each animal went its own way. Friendships grew up within the community and changed from time to time ; but alliances were formed when, for example, they had to punish one or

I

other of the animals. Friends shared their stores of food, handing portions of it to each other. They all united immediately to attack a new-comer. The chimpanzees very seldom clasped hands in greeting one another, but often did so in order to express their sense of good fellowship in particularly enjoyable situations. In more effusive greetings, gestures were made distinctly suggestive of sexual emotion. A favourite form of greeting was to stretch out the arm with the paw curved inwards ; this gesture was used as a sign of welcome, and was extended to friendly human beings to whom they were attached, and to other apes ; it was also used in the recognition of their own photographs. Chimpanzees regard a friendly human being as belonging to their group.

If a chimpanzee was isolated for experimental purposes it behaved as though it had gone out of its senses ; the remainder of the group showed much less excitement over the loss of their companion. The same sort of thing happened when after the lapse of a few weeks the imprisoned chimpanzee returned from its isolation. This differed, however, with the ape concerned. If it was the oldest animal, which invariably held a special position in the community, the rejoicings were always greater than in the case of one of the younger apes.

One or other of the chimpanzees was sometimes shut up in a cage by itself ; although it always howled and moaned, its companions did not come immediately to the cage and embrace it : thereupon it would stretch imploring arms towards them, and if they still did not come it would push its blanket, straw, or any other movable object in the cage, between the bars and brandish it in the air, but always in the direction of the other chimpanzees, finally throwing the objects, one after another, towards them.

Playthings, such as jam tins, pieces of wood, stones, rags, etc., were often carried about wedged between the lower part of the stomach and the upper part of the thigh. By way of greeting they sometimes put their hands in each other's laps, or one would take the hand of the other and draw it into its own lap. The animals were inclined to use this form of greeting without hesitation in their intercourse with men, thus recognizing them as friends and beings of a nature resembling their own. Köhler denies that this ceremony has a sexual origin ; believing rather that the apes press the hand of a friend into the place where they are accustomed to hide their treasures. Whether the action is purely instinctive (i.e. whether it is carried out by chimpanzees in their natural state), or whether it was invented by one of the captive animals and imitated by the others is not known.

If a chimpanzee climbs up its keeper in order to reach some object, and the keeper then bends down so that the attempt does not succeed, it will try to induce the keeper to straighten himself. If the animals need water they will drag the keeper with all the force at their disposal to the door behind which the water butt is usually kept. If some object is out of reach they will persuade a man to approach them and then take his hand and move it in the required direction. In consequence of the close morphological similarity between apes and men, apes find it easy to understand the nature of the human body.

The chimpanzees were capable of taking each other's part, or the part of their keepers, against other men or other chimpanzees. After quarrelling they always showed a strong desire for reconciliation. Jealousy was an emotion by no means unknown among them. An animal would plead not only for itself but for another, before punishment. According to von Oertzen, a young gorilla will also, before being punished, try to cajole its keeper. Chimpanzees embrace one another and also human beings as a sign of affection, or when they are frightened ; and these embraces are accompanied by a stroking of the back.

According to Köhler chimpanzees communicate with one another by means of noises and gestures, but neither noise nor gesture could be interpreted as the designation of an object.

Many of their gestures and sounds could be understood by human beings without difficulty, but some remained obscure. On the other hand the chimpanzees always understood each other immediately. Laughing and weeping is unknown among them, and they are always at a loss when confronted with human laughter.

The behaviour of a mother and child in captivity during the first three months of a young chimpanzee's life has been described by von Allesch. At first the other chimpanzees took a deep interest in the newly born infant, but afterwards their interest faded. The mother, as far as she could, avoided all excitement, and tried, for instance, to soothe another chimpanzee when it made a noise by patting it softly and caressingly.

The members of a society may be extremely attached to

one another.   This, for example, is said to be specially characteristic of bullfinches.   If one of a flock of these birds, collected together between two breeding seasons, is shot, the others remain near it for a long time, uttering cries of sorrow. This occurs more especially when the flock is small, that is to say when the birds stand in an unusually close relation to one another.   If two domesticated hens fall to fighting, the cock not infrequently separates them ; one cock may also intervene between two others which are fighting, but never does so unless it is superior to both the combatants.

It is not always possible to draw the line sharply between closed and open societies.   A brooding colony of penguins may certainly be classified, in general, as an open society, if only in virtue of the number of its members, and yet, as we have seen, each group of nests is a closed society.   In other cases our knowledge is still so incomplete that we do not know in which category to place our instances.   The mammals mentioned below, which live in colonies, are, therefore, included in this section only under reservations.

Members of the genus of marmots lay out subterranean dwelling places, and inhabit them in large numbers between one breeding season and another ; when these animals come to the surface of the ground they post sentinels.

Among vizcacha the subterranean dwelling of one animal will be connected by passages with those of several others. Settlements of this kind are called vizcachera. Within them there seems to be always one old male which assumes the rôle of leader.   Neighbouring settlements are linked by well-trodden paths used by the animals for visiting one another.

If a vizcachera is destroyed, the inmates are rescued by the inhabitants of the neighbouring colonies.

In Germany beavers are now usually found living in pairs ; only in the most retired localities do they still form colonies, whether large or small. In more populous regions they usually house themselves in simple subterranean burrows, and do not build a fort. These forts, when they do occur, are oven-shaped, thick-walled mounds, made of peeled sticks and branches, earth, clay and sand, and they contain an inner living room, and a chamber used for storing food. In places where the animals are left undisturbed a large number will toil together at building a fort. The females are the real architects and builders, while the males collect and furnish the necessary materials. If the water changes its level in the course of the year, or is not of sufficient depth, the beavers build a dam across the stream and stem its flow. The dams are built of the same material as that used for the fort, and have an almost vertical wall on the water front, but on the other side merely an escarpment. Any breaches in the dam are sought out and repaired. Canadian beavers sometimes support an original dam with others built out from the base of the first. The dams of European and Canadian beavers are said to be hundreds of years old, and if this is true then countless generations must have laboured on them and toiled for their preservation.

Animals belonging to species which, under natural conditions, have no intercourse with one another, will make friends in captivity, driven thereto by the lack of any other outlet for their gregarious impulses. An ape may become genuinely attached to a sheep, a pig, a rabbit, a parrot, or a bird of prey ; and captive animals very often quickly develop an affection for their keepers. Schillings was able to increase the happiness of a young, newly caught rhinoceros very considerably by giving it the companionship of a full-grown female goat. Friendly relations were established between the animals in the course of a very few days, although neither of them derived any material profit from the presence of the other ; the goat did not, for instance, suckle the young rhinoceros. The friendship became, indeed, so close, that the goat often disposed itself for sleep leaning against the rhinoceros. Tame baboons, like some dogs, are devoted only to their masters, greeting them joyfully, but showing themselves invariably hostile and ill-tempered towards strangers. A caged marabout would greet Schillings by flapping its wings and nodding its head, and would not rest content until its master had caressed it. Although this marabout would have nothing to do with any other animal in Schillings' camp, it was on terms of close friendship with a young rhinoceros.

Brehm, from his own experience of chimpanzees, judges that in their intercourse with men they subordinate themselves to higher talents and powers, whereas they regard other animals with the same consciousness of superiority as that with which men regard them. Chimpanzees always behave with great gentleness towards children, having a special affection for the smallest. Brehm believes that this indicates that the anthropoid apes recognize man, the superior, even in the smallest child. They comport themselves with much less consideration towards their own kind, more especially when they are younger than themselves.

In the common ape cage in the Berlin aquarium a young
gorilla treats only a young chimpanzee as its equal, choosing
it alone as a companion to play with and caress, and behaving
with a complete lack of consideration towards the other
non-anthropoid apes.

Brehm describes a friendship between two full-grown apes,
a long-tailed monkey and a baboon. The long-tailed monkey
was completely dominated by the very much larger baboon,
it would not venture abroad nor take food except in the
company of the latter. If the monkey did not voluntarily
share his food with the baboon the latter would use force,
sometimes even extracting morsels from the cheek pouches
of the other, and it was very seldom seen to reverse the
procedure by giving something to the monkey. According
to the same author, a small ape, kept captive on a ship,
when it was to be punished would take refuge on the breast
of an orang utan, and the orang utan would then climb with
it into the rigging, against its usual habit, and remain there
until the danger was past.

Schillings relates how, in a fort in East Africa, a friendship
grew up between an old captive male baboon and a small
native child about a year and a half old. Each day, from its
hut near by, the child would crawl to the ape and play with
it for several hours.

Caged parrots may form intimate friendships with one
another, even when they belong to different species. If a
male and a female are shut up together amorous relations
often develop between them and the birds will bill together
hour after hour ; it sometimes happens, in fact, that if one
of them dies the other does not long survive. According to

Brehm, a captive purple water-hen (*Porphyrio*) assumed the attitude of the sexual act both in the presence of its keeper and of a lory. The lory frequently attempted coition, and attacked the keeper, screeching if he stroked the purple water-hen.

It may here be mentioned that, under natural conditions, the weaver-bird (*Dinemellia dinemelli*) lives in intimate relation on the one hand with *Spreo superbus*, and on the other with the great grey shrike (Schillings). These birds play together in the air, chase each other as butterflies do, perch close to one another, etc.

2 The Open Society

The characteristic feature of an open society is that, as compared with a closed society, it is much less exclusive. Chance alone determines whether its members shall come together or separate ; but when they do unite social ties of various kinds are formed immediately ; in particular, the animals concerned act with conspicuous uniformity (e.g. in flight, foraging, resting, etc.). If, in such open societies, any hierarchy is established, if watches are set during the resting periods, and leaders come forward, the community becomes (*a*) an organized open society ; if, however, the community is homogeneous in the sense that apart from chance differences of size and strength no one member is superior to another, then it is (*b*) an unorganized open society.

a *The Organized Open Society*

The herds and bands of mammals which gather together between two pairing seasons are often open, and yet organized, societies. One animal acts as leader, and it is common for watches to be set while the herd rests. Herds of gnus and buffaloes often rest on hills dominating the surrounding country (von Oertzen). Herds of. giraffes are led either by a male or a female, and this also is true of herds of cow antelopes. In the latter sentinels often take up their stand upon anthills.

According to Pallas (quoted by Brehm) the saiga antelope lives in large herds ; the old males remain with the herd throughout the year. Single animals are always on guard, and no sentinel ever betakes itself to rest without calling upon another animal, by nodding to it and advancing towards it in a peculiar manner, to relieve it. Only when another animal has risen to its feet and taken over the watch does the first one lie down. These antelopes, when danger threatens, first herd together, and then take flight in a long line led generally by a male, but sometimes by a female.

In other species the leader is either always a male or always a female. Among wild reindeer, it is the leader, a female, which invariably acts as sentry and remains standing even when all the other members of the herd are resting ; if it signifies its intention to lie down, another female immediately rises to its feet. If danger is near the leader may induce the rest of the herd to rise to their feet by prodding the animals with its horns. In certain circumstances, as is well known, a herd of animals will follow its leader blindly, even when the latter precipitates itself into an abyss. If the leader is killed the herd may lose its head completely. Herds of Caing whales are also led by old males, whom they are said to follow blindly. Brehm relates that one of these whales, which escaped when the rest of its herd was massacred by coast-dwellers, returned again and again to its dead and dying companions.

In a herd of cattle the leading cow possesses the largest bell. The cattle recognize exactly the tinklings made by the bells of their own herd, and usually find their way back to the herd again after straying. The leader displays a certain feeling of rank, and will not allow another animal to precede it. In South America large herds of llamas are used as beasts of burden and the leader is a male richly decked with blankets. Similarly the leader of a South American caravan of mules is always sumptuously adorned. Among sheep, a leader furnished with a bell keeps a flock of three to four thousand head together. If the bell ceases to sound the flock breaks up into groups of six to twelve sheep, each with its own leader. The action of man in making one selected animal recognizable at long range, enables it to act as leader to several thousands of its own kind. I have myself observed among the goats living at the edge of the Zillertal forest, that the leader provided with the bell does not, in every case, guide the herd, and that consequently the remaining animals sometimes do not imitate its movements. The leader is often to be found in the centre of the herd; the animals which happen to be in the front ranks determine in which direction the herd shall move, and the leader is, so to speak carried along with the stream. In such cases, the leader forms rather a rallying point, from which none of the animals stray very far.

Schjelderup-Ebbe has shown how an order of precedence comes into existence within societies. A flock of fowls in a fowl run is not exclusive in the sense that its members make common cause against a new arrival, leaving the latter isolated. The new-comer may safely attach itself to the flock, but the position it is to hold therein must first be won by fighting. For no two hens ever live side by side in a flock without having previously settled, either for the time being, or for good, which is the superior and which the inferior ; the " pecking order " thus established decides which of the birds may peck the other without fear of being pecked in return. Similar pecking codes exist, according to Schjelderup-Ebbe, among sparrows, wild ducks, and possibly among many other kinds of animals. Pecking among cocks is governed by the same rules as among hens, except that the cocks exhibit greater ferocity. Such " pecking orders " give the society concerned a certain degree of organization.

Sometimes the " pecking order " results in a continuous list being formed ; that is to say, one hen pecks all the others, the next in order pecks all but the first, and so on, down to the humblest member of the community which is pecked by all the rest of the flock. But it may happen that three hens peck one another, so to speak, in triangular order, i.e. A pecks B, B pecks C, but C pecks A ; or the order may be a quadrilateral sequence of the kind $A \rightarrow B \rightarrow C \rightarrow D \rightarrow A$. This is enough to prove that strength alone is not the deciding factor. A hen low on the list is usually much more cruel to the remaining hens which it may peck than a hen which occupies a higher rank. The hen which is entitled to peck all the others is generally the least malicious. A threatening note usually precedes the pecking and is often sufficient by itself to put the offender to flight.

Which of two hens is to be the inferior and which the superior is settled, as a rule, at the first encounter ; one of the hens may yield without a struggle, or the issue may have to be fought out. The triangular and quadrilateral arrangements which occur within the " pecking order " are explained by the fact that the hens sometimes submit without fighting. Not infrequently the stronger hens allow themselves to be pecked by the weaker. The reason is that the younger hens are usually attacked by the older, the new-comers by the established residents, and the sick by the healthy, and the order, once established, is permanent. If several weak hens simultaneously attack a stronger one and defeat it, the latter is afterwards pecked by each of the former. Katz and Toll tested the intelligence of different fowls, and have established that the fowl which stands at the head of the list is also the most intelligent, and that, roughly, the position within the social scale corresponds to ascertained differences of intelligence.

The tendency to form a social organization is innate in quite young chickens, whether or not they have been brought up with older fowls; it follows that the tendency must be purely instinctive and in no way dependent upon tradition. I think one can go even further and say that the instinct is, in a measure, indispensable to the very existence of social life among such animals (which, unlike the state-building insects, live mainly for themselves, and not for the welfare of the " state "). If this instinct failed immediately to establish a recognized order, such animals would pass their lives in a state of constant warfare, since their social instincts prompt them to seek one another's company, while their self-assertive instincts urge them continually to attack one another. The " pecking order " is of great importance to the hens, for the superior bird is not disturbed when on the nest, nor robbed of its food, whereas it may disturb others and infringe their rights with impunity. The battles between hens or cocks are, therefore, not mere sport. A cock wields, in every case, despotic sway over all the hens, and will often interfere between two fighting hens,or even between two cocks which are attacking one another (provided, in this case, he is the superior of both the combatants). With penguins the case is different ; for if the males fall to fighting, the females sometimes throw themselves between the antagonists and separate them.

The position of a hen on the " pecking list " is occasionally altered as the result of a fight ; in such cases it is an oppressed hen which revolts against her oppressor. Such a rebellion occurs less frequently when the position was initially decided by fighting than when it was tacitly accepted. A battle of this kind either confirms the previous state of affairs or reverses it. A hen revolting against the hitherto recognized superior fights less fiercely than at other times ; this proves the existence of a psychic obstacle to such an attack.

Once a hen has fallen into an inferior position, it is more difficult for it to mutiny and thereby gain superiority, than if it had fought for its place from the outset.

During breeding time a hen shows itself much more easily irritated by other hens, and not infrequently revolts against its superiors. A hen with chickens is full of courage ; but if the chickens are taken away, even for a short time, this courage vanishes and the hen allows itself to be attacked and overcome by any aggressor (compare here the case of the male stickleback robbed of its nest).

If two flocks of fowls are penned together, flock does not fight flock, but as time goes on a series of single combats take place. Behaviour of this kind must be regarded as characteristic of an open, and at the same time organized, society.

A recognized order of precedence also exists in a flock of wild ducks. Within any such flock, inhabiting some particular pond, it is agreed, both among the males and among the females, which is to be superior, which inferior. For every one of the birds recognizes every other with unfailing certainty (as is probably always the case among birds and mammals). Any male is superior to every female. The battles fought for social superiority are never as fierce among wild ducks as among domestic fowls. The winner is thenceforward entitled to bite, whereas the former must always submit to being bitten.

Some bird societies show a more advanced type of organization in that they set guards and send out scouts. Thus flocks of cranes (which may be composed of different species), in their winter quarters, are guarded while at rest by sentinels. If a flock has been disturbed in any given place, before it returns to the neighbourhood again scouts are sent ahead to spy out the land. Flamingoes set guards at night ; if these are killed noiselessly it is possible to kill many of the remaining flamingoes while they are still asleep. Flocks of geese and flocks of parrots safeguard themselves while resting by posting sentinels. Crows also set guards while the flock is feeding. Cockatoos out on a marauding expedition send scouts ahead of the main flock. A certain stage oɪ organization can be inferred from the fact that during migration the separate species always observe a special flight formation.

Leaders, too, occur among birds; thus, among the *Penelope* species the birds gather between two breeding seasons in flocks containing from sixty to eighty head, under the leadership of an old male. In a flock made up of different species the largest bird is often the leader; for example, sometimes in the winter a gathering of titmice, nut-hatches, and creepers will be led by a great-spotted woodpecker.

A flock of sleeping partridges provides an instance of the organization of a whole society, for they pass the night in a circle with their heads turned outwards; a herd of wild swine on the contrary so arrange themselves for sleeping that every head is turned towards the centre of the ring.

The members of some species of animals join together to form more or less organized hunting packs. Wolves live during the winter in packs; a pack of this kind travels in single file, one animal treading in the footsteps made by another in the snow. The animals hunt in common, and the pack divides into two bodies, one of which pursues the prey while the other bars its path. The African hyæna (*Lycaon*) hunts in packs for large game. The animals in the rear follow the chord of the arcs described by the animals in front, relieve these latter at the point of intersection, and take the lead themselves; this manœuvre being repeated until the prey is exhausted. Lions hunt together where the country is rich in game, at times accompanied by their young ; some act as beaters, others capture the prey ; while on the hunt, their roars appear to have some important significance. According to von Oertzen three tame young leopards combined to hunt fowls ; one drove the birds while the other two ambushed them. I have already mentioned the case of the dogs rendered masterless by the Russian invasion of East Prussia in 1915, which, in their distress formed packs of about a dozen and hunted in open formation across the fields.

A pair of birds of prey will often hunt together, each mate helping the other. Marabout (*Leptoptilos*) hunt in flocks on the grassy plains of South Africa for the numerous grasshoppers to be found there, allying themselves often with storks in this pursuit. The birds spread themselves into a far-flung line, and move in this formation over the open ground, thus beating a wide area. Gannets fly side by side in a long string in their pursuit of flying fishes. Screamers fly over water together in large flocks, and from time to time a number of the birds dive down to fish. Pelicans fish together in shallow waters. They form a circle, and then narrow it slowly by swimming towards one another, or they make a semi-circle and advance towards the shore. In rivers they form two lines which advance towards each other. Cormorants are said to fish together sometimes systematically, in a sheet of water or over a particular stretch of the sea, in just the same way as pelicans. But among the birds I have named (marabouts, storks, gannets, screamers, pelicans, cormorants) mutual assistance (i.e. if one calls by this name their hunting in common) is never carried to the point of mutual defence.

b The Unorganized Open Society

The migrating societies formed by many, strictly speaking, non-social insects, which at certain times collect in swarms and travel together over the ground or through the air, are unorganized societies (grass-hoppers, dragon-flies, butter-flies, caterpillars, etc.). The permanent associations formed by certain kinds of caterpillars must likewise be named unorganized societies.

I had occasion to observe in the aquarium of the Biological Institute in Heligoland how a swarm of animals may act uniformly, even though it is moving forward without a leader. Large and small *Ammodytes* live there in mixed swarms ; these two species rarely swim along with mackerel, but when this happens, the mackerel, as the larger fish, always lead the way. Assuming that a swarm of *Ammodytes* are swimming in a straight line across the tank and one of the fishes suddenly makes a turn, its example is immediately followed by another. According to whether most, or, ultimately all the others follow the lead thus given, the swarm as a whole swerves aside from the initial direction ; or else those fishes which had swerved aside reverse their movements and return to the main swarm as it proceeds on its way. It is certain that these animals keep together chiefly by the help of sight ; for when a swarm completely reverses its direction, one fish will turn to the left and another to the right, which would not occur if they were guided by a sense of taste or vibrations set up in the water. If one of the swarm falls behind or deviates, temporarily, from the path of its companions, it forthwith tries to regain the swarm by accelerating its movements, and the necessary turns are so promptly and surely carried out that they must be guided by sight alone. Even when *Ammodytes* and mackerel are swimming apart, the former may readily leave their original course to follow the latter. On the other hand, solitary fishes remain totally unaffected by alterations in the movements of other fishes.

Among the highest species of molluscs, some, like the Cephalopods (cuttlefish), live a genuinely gregarious life ; swarms of them may migrate over great distances. In the aquarium one can observe how the whole mass, like a real swarm of fishes, changes its direction simultaneously. Likewise, certain reptiles live in societies (lizards, geckos, agamas, chameleons, etc.), which do not, however, seem to possess any social grading or any real organization.

Some fishes, among them salmon and herrings, are reported to travel in V or wedge formation. In the case of the latter the larger and stronger fish are said to form the van, which would seem to indicate the existence of a certain rudimentary type of organization. Shoals of herrings are, likewise, divided according to the generations to which the fishes belong. If a shoal is scattered, as a rule it speedily reunites. Whether or not the shoals keep together during the night is disputed. In some species the bond uniting individuals is so close that when one fish discovers a way of escape from the net all the others follow instantly.

It has been observed among sticklebacks and other species that some one individual, whether male or female, is specially feared by its companions, which it constantly attacks and drives away, particularly when feeding. If it turns out that in swarms of this kind superiority is accorded to greater biting powers, such swarms should not come under the present heading, but should rank as organized societies.

At breeding time, as I have described, the male sticklebacks desert the swarm, and each one takes possession of a special domain which it defends against intruders. By way of experiment a large fish which preys upon sticklebacks was placed in a tank containing a number of males of the latter species. These, which had hitherto kept to themselves, each in its own domain, immediately united again with each other, and with the females, into a swarm ; so that in face of a superior enemy their gregarious instincts reasserted themselves. The same behaviour is reported (Brehm) of the American oriole. Each pair defends its particular domain against its neighbours, but a cry of fear will bring the latter out instantly to do battle with the common enemy.

VIII GENERAL ANIMAL SOCIOLOGY (*continued*)

B MUTUAL HELP AND MUTUAL HARM

Mutual help in the animal kingdom, and its contrary, mutual harm, form a much disputed section of animal sociology (see particularly Kropotkin). Cases of mutual assistance occur frequently ; it would be folly to deny them. But it is unwise to generalize too freely from these occurrences, or to regard them from a sentimental point of view. For it is also a fact that mutual harm plays a large part in the animal world, not only between members of the same species, but even between members of the same society.

The most obvious type of mutual help consists in one animal, though not itself attacked, hurrying to intervene on behalf of another on hearing a cry, either of warning, or of fear. Schultz relates that when one of his young rhinoceroses was attacked it, in turn, immediately assumed the offensive, while the other hurried forward to take part in the fray. Among Köhler's chimpanzees, if one was exposed to a real or feigned attack all the rest hastened to assist in its defence. Thus every ape enjoys the protection of all the remaining members of the horde ; should any beast of prey attack one of them, every able-bodied member of the horde hurls itself against the aggressor (unless the assailant possesses obviously overpowering strength). It is universally related of apes that they carry wounded or dead companions away with them ; according to Brehm, a mother baboon has even been seen to pluck leaves from the nearest branch and use them to stop a wound inflicted upon her offspring. In case of danger one animal often warns another, and according to Berger a Patas monkey once tried to prevent its master from touching a box which contained a snake (it must, however, be stated that the snake was dead). It may also be mentioned that prairie marmots and vizcachas drag their wounded companions back to their burrows, and even alligators lend assistance to wounded members of their own species If a vizcachera is overthrown its inmates are dug out by their neighbours.

According to Berger (p. 225), the instinct to help a sick companion is stronger in elephants than in any other species of animal, with the exception of apes. If an elephant is wounded by a bullet others come forward and support it ; if it falls its fellows kneel by it, and some pass their tusks under its body while others wind their trunks about its neck and attempt to put it on its feet.

The members of a horde of apes search one another's coats for burrs and thorns after a flight. This habit must not be confused with that of hunting for lice, which the apes commonly practise upon one another, but which they will practise upon men, if allowed to do so. Brehm interprets the habit (vol. 13, p. 436) not as a search for vermin (and not, therefore, as a form of mutual assistance), but as prompted by a taste for licking the small salt particles of skin which peel from the body (i.e. as a form of self-indulgence). It has been proved that the skin parasites escape unharmed.

Members of most animal societies display jealousy of their companions over questions of food (apes, beasts of prey, etc.), though it is true that two apes, close friends of one another, will share their food. The most conspicuous feature of the behaviour of hens in a flock of fowls is jealousy ; the cock alone remains indifferent to their brawls ; he exercises despotic sway over every hen, and even entices them to any spot where food happens to be particularly plentiful.

Mutual help very often occurs in connexion with pairing and brood tending. The male protects the female, and either one or both of the parents defend the offspring. Young animals which have lost their mother are sometimes immediately adopted by another female (e.g. among elephants, wild pigs, quails, and some ducks). It is well known that the maternal instinct in cats is so strongly developed that one can impose upon them the young of widely different species, namely, young rats, mice, rabbits, hares, dogs, foxes, squirrels, etc. According to Brehm, some parrots, when kept in captivity, take over the care of young or crippled birds of their own species or even of animals of a different race, feeding them and defending them against aggression. As we shall see later, however, this does not always happen, and it is even possible for the contrary to occur.

Female apes, too, when kept in captivity, will grudge food to their own offspring ; the nature of the environment, which is always unfavourable, though in varying degrees, is probably responsible for this behaviour. Foster children, adopted to satisfy the maternal instinct, are especially liable to suffer from this behaviour. Sometimes, even, they are altogether refused access to the food.

It cannot be denied that apes possess a certain tendency to cruelty. We must nevertheless be particularly careful when discussing this topic ; for much which may seem at first sight to proceed from an instinct of cruelty—an instinct which makes torture an end in itself—on closer examination proves to be bound up with the biological necessities of the species concerned. Thus it is highly debateable whether a full-grown cat playing with a mouse affords an instance of deliberate cruelty ; quite possibly, the cat is simply keeping in practice. This is certainly the correct interpretation when a mother cat carries to its young a half-dead mouse for them to practise on. But whoever reflects on the impossibility of disentangling the skein of human motives, will hardly deny that, in the play of the full-grown cat, there may be a sort of sport and will-to-power. Many intermediate stages exist, nevertheless, between this latter impulsion and genuine cruelty.

The games which even full-grown apes will play together are not always quite harmless, especially when some of the players are stronger than others. Apes often show a propensity to tug a companion unexpectedly by the tail or by the hair. In every monkey cage each animal occupies a clearly defined rank, and the larger ones will tease and torment those of a smaller species in every conceivable way, seizing them, for instance, by the tail to send them flying through the air. Yerkes (1916, p. 121) noticed a young ape gleefully inciting his companions against one another. The animal in question pretended to have been attacked by another ape ; as soon as the elder ones had come to blows, it withdrew to a safe distance and watched developments. Brehm describes how a baboon teased a dog by pulling its tail and then running away, repeating the trick until the dog was beside itself with fury. Apes are particularly fond of chasing and intimidating fowls. In considering these cases it must, however, be remembered that the apes being in captivity are, so to speak, condemned to idleness. They are cut off from all the normal activities which they pursue in a state of freedom, and their energy has to seek an outlet in other directions.

When in Köhler's experiments, the apes piled two or three boxes on top of one another in order to reach food hung above their heads, although they helped each other to do this, their actions were prompted rather by their common anxiety to get at the food than by any more altruistic motive. Ordinarily they were far more inclined to hinder than to help one another. When one of the animals was at work, perched high upon a rickety erection, the unoccupied chimpanzees would steal up behind and give the boxes a vigorous push, thus upsetting the whole structure and bringing the worker to the ground ; they would then make off with all possible speed.

A sick or wounded animal is often turned out of a society, i.e. ostracised, or even killed. Alpine marmots gather together before going into their winter quarters and, according to Girtaner, it sometimes happens then that a number of them attack, and bite to death, an old and decrepit comrade. The biological significance of such a " weeding-out " is obvious, for if one of the animals dies during hibernation the corpse is a danger to the whole community. Beavers have been seen to bite and drive out of their colonies certain of their fellows, both young and old. Animals thus expelled live thenceforth alone in a separate structure. Many tales have been told of the so-called " stork tribunals ", and " executions " among other animals. The following, however, is ascertained truth. A number of cranes have often been seen to fall upon one bird while the flock is resting, and inflict such severe blows upon it with their beaks as to lame or even kill it. Storks collect in large flocks before migrating, and expel or even kill those which are sick or incapable of making the journey, or which have been tamed by human beings. Ravens, cranes, and many other birds, hares and roebuck show themselves hostile to tame members of their own species (Naumann, vol. vi, p. 305 ; vol. vii, p. 104). Many birds will not suffer the presence of companions with gun-shot wounds, but kill them outright. Brehm relates that a parrot, after being wounded, was ostracised by its companions ; it then lived alone until it was put to death by some other parrots. The " execution " of single animals is occasionally met with among many beasts of prey, and even among domestic cattle ; Gross (p. 228) is of the opinion that not all these cases are to be explained as the working of an instinct having as its object the preservation of the species ; it would be sufficient for this purpose merely to expel any animal whose presence endangered the life of the community and leave it to its fate ; he thinks them often due rather to an instinct of destruction.

Cannibalism, or the killing and devouring of each other by members of the same species, is of frequent occurrence in the animal kingdom. For this, of course, one of the creatures must get a hold on the other ; the animal attacked must therefore be either the weaker of the two, or somehow prevented from defending itself. Among solitary predatory species (worms and other of the lower animals, insects, crayfish, reptiles, birds of prey, shrew-mice, predatory mammals), animals belonging to the same species never spare one another ; e.g. the male hamster even bites the female to death if they encounter one another outside the breeding season, without, it is true, troubling itself further about the corpse. Some species even devour their own offspring ; in particular, the parent which does not concern itself with the rearing of the brood is a danger to its own young (fishes, crocodiles, predatory mammals) ; among fishes, however, the parent which does tend the brood may devour its young after they have reached a certain size. The male budgerigar, which helps its mate to feed the young birds as long as they are in the nest, sometimes ill-treats and even kills them after they are fledged. Similarly, unmated female budgerigars are also a source of danger to young birds of their own species. Parent ostriches bite and kill the offspring of other birds ; among gallinaceous birds the females peck to death chickens belonging to other hens; unmated ostrich hens do the same and half-grown ostriches deal similarly with younger members of their own species ; the turkey-cock kills his own young. In exceptional cases, ostriches driven from their nest will destroy their own offspring. The biological significance of such behaviour escapes us.

Cephalopods (cuttlefish), living under natural conditions,

eat one another ; if, for instance, one of a number is hooked
by a fisherman, its companions immediately seize upon it,
and may even allow themselves to be drawn to the surface
clinging to its body. Caged owls live peaceably together
as long as they are all equally strong and healthy, but if
one falls sick it is immediately attacked and eaten by its
companions ; and this holds true even when the owls
come from one and the same nest. If a musk rat, a brown
rat, or a water rat is caught in a trap it is torn to pieces
alive, and devoured by its fellows. To pinch the tail of
a caged rat until it squeaks with pain is sometimes enough
to induce its fellow prisoners to fall upon it and bite it
to death.

The mutual help which is a feature of the life of an insect
state has already been described. As I have said, the
habit of licking each other must be regarded, not as due to
a desire for cleanliness, but rather as a means of procuring
the skin secretions which are the object of the licking.
But there is a limit to mutual help in these insect states ;
whilst it remains true that under certain conditions sick
and wounded ants are tended and licked, they are just as
frequently left uncared-for, or carried off to the rubbish
heap. Sentiment plays no part in the organization of these
states ; only those insects which work for, or will in future
work for the state, are tended and protected ; the common-
weal alone determines life or death. Here again let it be
emphasized that neither intelligent reflection nor a majority
of votes govern insect states, but sureness of instinct and
the limitations of instincts to specific purposes, things
which appear fabulous to us as human beings.

Any individual belonging to another nest, or lacking the special nest odour, is put to death. The queen bee kills all rivals; once the queen has been fecundated the workers expel the henceforth superfluous males from the hive. Queen ants also commonly fight one another until only one remains alive. If times are hard the worker ants may kill every queen but one (Escherich, p. 86). Many of the eggs are eaten by the ants, an insect often eating those it has laid itself. Termite workers take good care that the numerical proportions of the " castes " are correct ; superfluous insects are killed and eaten (Escherich, p. 22) ; a similar fate overtakes their dead or diseased comrades.

C THE COLLECTIVE MIND

Mass psychology, as is well-known, proves the truth of the dictum that the whole is not merely the sum of the parts. In other words, the collective effect, obtained by the cooperation of individuals, can never be inferred from the mere summation of individual achievements. Thus the mass, or collective action M, cannot be ascertained by adding together the single actions of the individuals, A, B, C; their co-operation produces a result *sui generis*. The equation then is not :—

$$M = f(A) + f(B) + f(C)$$

but—

$$M = f(A, B, C).$$

The importance of the individual in contributing to the collective result depends upon the part it plays in the community. In certain cases the individual determines the life or death of the whole community, as, for instance, in the case of a bell wether jumping into an abyss.

Among social species courage and pugnacity grow in proportion to the number of individuals present ; this is true of ants, bees, humble bees, wasps, hornets, and others. In the case of the honey bee, a small and weak community often does not defend itself against enemies which it could easily repulse, whereas a strong community is always ready for attack, and expels every intruder (*v.* Buttel-Reepen). According to Forel, one and the same ant which is full of courage among its fellows will take to flight before a much weaker adversary as soon as it finds itself alone. State-building insects are overcome by profound depression if their nest disappears.

Song birds, and other small birds, when united, " tease " birds of prey, i.e. defend themselves to the best of their ability against them, not only in our own country, but in other lands and latitudes. Single sea-gulls and crows are powerless against many kinds of enemies ; but, united, the members of a colony of crows or a colony of sea-gulls often wage war against birds of prey. A herd of horses or domestic swine will attack a wolf, whereas a solitary horse or pig is generally lost. In the same way wolves are much bolder when hunting in a pack than when hunting alone.

When many individuals are together the action of a few sometimes carries away the whole group. In warm weather, a large number of locusts sitting closely packed together gradually become more and more excited ; until suddenly they all take flight together, attracting to their ranks every member of their own species they overtake so that the swarm grows larger and larger. (Brehm, vol. ii, p. 96.) Migrating swarms of dragon-flies are formed in this way, as are the swarms of locust larvæ which travel across the ground. Similarly among ants the excitement of the males and females preparing for the nuptial flight communicates itself to the workers, and no work is done until the last of them has flown. According to Stresemann a flock of birds increases because of the fascination exercised on the individual by the mass; sometimes even a pair of birds leading a solitary life will be carried away by the spell.

Köhler noticed that if one of his chimpanzees was attacked the whole group immediately hastened to its aid. During a fight the animals would scream themselves into ever-increasing fury. Sometimes a single cry of indignation was sufficient to set the whole band in an uproar, although perhaps the majority of the animals had seen nothing of the original cause of the trouble, which might have been either a genuine attack or a mere misunderstanding.

Panics frequently take place among social animals. Tame doves may be thrown into a panic during the night if one of their number happens to flap its wings (Whitman). The half wild horses of South America are sometimes seized with panic. Hundreds and thousands will suddenly take madly to their heels, cast themselves against rocks and precipitate themselves into chasms. Any carriage or saddle horse belonging to travellers who happen to be resting near is drawn into their flight. Sheep take madly to flight before wolves, and, in Australia, before the wild dogs (dingoes) of the country, straying so far afield that they often perish. Schillings relates the following anecdote of an old male baboon chained in front of a fort in East Africa. On one occasion the whole black population of the station, expecting at any moment to be attacked by enemy tribes, fled to take refuge in the fort ; the baboon, seeing this, tore itself from its chain and fled with them to shelter.

Some actions are performed with much greater energy when they are carried out by a group of individuals ; this is notoriously true of singing and dancing, both among men and beasts. It is also true of gregarious animals when they are feeding ; farmers know that some beasts, e.g. horses and pigs, especially when young, eat more if fed with their companions. I have even heard a human mother say that it was better for her children to have a table-companion as otherwise they ate too little In all these cases we observe the working of that instinct which lies at the root of the pleasure taken by adult human beings in banqueting and other social entertainments.

D Courtship and Dancing

At pairing time more or less serious battles develop between the males for the possession of the females, not, it is true, among lower animals, but among the arthropods and the vertebrata. These are accompanied by a display of those arts by which one sex seeks to please the other ; rivalries between males at times constitute an art of wooing. It sometimes happens that the fighting loses its original significance and is no longer undertaken solely in order to dispose of a rival but becomes an end in itself ; in this case the battle becomes a sport, which may be serious or quite innocent. Finally the bodily movements, originally employed either in fighting or in wooing, may become freed from all sexual meaning and so conventionalized as no longer to express anything more than a sense of enhanced vitality.

Among insects male stag beetles sometimes fight to the death, as do also male ground wasps, solitary bees, and others. Male fishes often fight each other fiercely ; the victor disports himself amorously before the female, or they dally together for a while until eventually the female lays her eggs and the male immediately fertilizes them. The fighting fish *Betta* is so markedly pugnacious that in Siam the natives match them together for sport. Male amphibians fight with less ferocity, in fact, they do little more than jostle one another. Male reptiles, on the contrary, may be much fiercer, as also some birds and mammals.

The characteristic features of the courtship and pairing of many species of birds and mammals are well-known. On the whole the male is more striking, stronger and more aggressive, and does the fighting and the wooing, while the female plays a more passive part. Among *turnices* and *phaleropes*, however, the females are more brilliantly coloured and larger than the males, they alone play and dispute over the possession of the males, and the male undertakes the rearing of the brood single-handed. Among pheasants it is rather the females which seek the favour of the males than *vice versa*. Among condors both sexes dance. The female bird emits a characteristic mating cry which obviously acts as a sexual stimulant upon the male, and among roes the " piping " of the females is an invitation to the male. Among human beings, too, we see that the female sex very seldom contents itself with playing a purely passive part.

L

The fighting principle is often carried to excess by some male birds and mammals. Thus, during pairing time, male chaffinches live in a state of constant hostility towards each other, either singing against one another or actually fighting, although this behaviour is quite uncalled for, since the females meanwhile sit in peace and unmolested in their nests. The tapping of the male woodpecker has the effect of attracting rivals ; this tapping is characteristic of the species in all latitudes, although it varies a little in different zones ; it might be described as instrumental music, and the woodpeckers of our own country produce the sound in this way ; the male suspends itself from a dry branch and taps it with his beak so hard and so quickly that the branch quivers to and fro : the noise of the hammering beak and the quivering branch together combine to produce the well-known rattle.

The battles which occur among stags at rutting time seem to be undertaken entirely for their own sake, for a stag on hearing the bellow of a rival will leave his harem in the lurch and set out to find the challenger. Here fighting has become a sport, though, as is well-known, such battles may have a fatal issue. Fights of this kind, but varying in severity, take place among many species of horned and antlered mammals, when the males are in heat. Bison steers, when frantic with desire, will root up comparatively large trees, and at rutting time one often finds both bulls and cows which they have killed.

Some birds play fighting games of a harmless nature. Among ruffs (*Machetes pugnax*), which mate promiscuously, during the spring the males collect every day at a certain spot to play the fighting game ; females seldom join them, but when they do appear they strike the attitudes of the male and pretend to join in the fray. In these fights, which although they appear to be very fierce, are never, in fact, serious, there is neither victor nor vanquished ; just outside the fighting ground several males are often to be seen keeping company peacefully with a single female, and no signs of real jealousy between males have ever been observed. The original biological importance of the fighting instinct has, in these cases, entirely disappeared.

In spite of the apparent ferocity with which black cocks attack one another on their dancing grounds, it hardly ever, perhaps never, happens that a bird is seriously wounded; among capercaillies, on the other hand, the males fight one another in earnest. Some black cock will visit several dancing grounds in the course of a single morning. In countries where black game is abundant, several cocks always appear simultaneously at a dancing place, where they fight each other and dance in each others' company ; fighting and dancing have become indistinguishable. The fight is just acted and serves no other purpose than to increase the sexual excitement of both males and females, and this may be affirmed in general of the fights, sports, wooings, and dances of birds.

White mews (*Rupicola*) play a kind of dancing game in which a male dances alone upon a piece of rock watched by a number of males and females perched upon the branches of bushes nearby. Each male dances in turn, and the females set up an outcry whenever one relieves another.

According to Hudson, certain South American giant rails

(*Aramides*) collect from time to time at fixed places and
perform a kind of pairing dance in which both sexes take
part (Doflein, fig. 383). The contagious effect of collective
performances turns these dances into " mass games of an
orgiastic nature " (Groos, p. 232). According to Groos, we
have here an instance of that stimulation of sexual
excitement by imitative suggestion with which ethnology
and the history of civilization have long since made us
familiar. Jacanas dance in the same way (Doflein, fig. 384).
According to Hudson, the South American spur-winged
peewit (*Belonopterus*) performs a dance which is so far
peculiar to that species that it is always performed by three
birds together (Doflein, illustration 385). This species lives
in pairs throughout the year ; but the different couples
keep close to one another and from time to time one of a
pair will visit a neighbouring couple, whereupon the dance is
immediately begun. The three birds fall into line one behind
the other, and march forward, keeping step and uttering
cries in time to their paces ; then they stop and the leading
bird stretches itself to its full height and sings loudly,
while the other two bow their heads and utter gentle notes.
After this the performance comes to an end, the visitor
returns to its mate and sooner or later receives a similar
visit. The existence of the winged spurs perhaps indicates
that the game was evolved from real fighting (Haecker).
Hudson believes that in the case of *Belonoptera* there is no
longer any connexion between this dance and the sexual
life of these birds, since the dance is performed at all seasons
of the year.

The males of different monogamous species of birds of

Paradise arrange dancing and pairing parties in special trees and at special times of the day when the breeding season begins. The trees to which the birds betake themselves then appear one mass of waving feathers ; the females are merely spectators of the proceedings.

At pairing time each male bower bird, helped by its mate builds on the ground a " playhouse " of twigs (Doflein, illustrations 386-9). This bower serves no other purpose than that of a theatre for their courtship, the actual nest being built in a tree. It has both a back and a front entrance, and is decked with all sorts of coloured or striking objects (feathers, shreds of cloth, snail shells and mussel shells, bleached bones, etc.) : the feathers being stuck among the twigs, and the bones and rags laid before the entrances These decorative objects are often brought from miles away. The bowers seem to be used several years in succession. In one species they are covered outside with long blades of grass laid neatly together. Carefully selected stones serve to keep the twigs and grasses in position. In this species, moreover, several males use the same bower. The gardener bird (*Amblyornis*) decks the space in front of its bower with coloured berries and flowers, and these, when faded, are thrown on a rubbish heap behind the bower and replaced by fresh ones. One particular male of a certain species was observed to drag a long, dead, and dried up centipede to the playing ground every day and wage with it a mock battle before the eyes of its mate and other birds.

Among the phenomena accompanying and succeeding pairing, when wooing time, in its strict sense, is already over, are many tricks of flying practised by the males, and sometimes by both sexes ; thus most of the larger birds of prey and also storks are accustomed in spring to fly in wide circles over the nesting places they have chosen.

Among cranes, which are birds of very high mental development, the dance has lost its wooing significance, and has become merely an expression of general well-being. Both males and females dance. The movements in this dance are executed for their own sake ; i.e. the birds play (Groos). " Demoiselle " cranes (*Grus virgo*) dance and play together in the following manner ; they collect on the steppes, form a circle, bow to one another, and dance in a fashion that is truly grotesque. Soon after pairing, too, they meet together morning and evening to dance and hop round each other, lifting their crests and their wings, and then fly around in wide circles. After a few weeks, when actual breeding begins, the birds cease to collect together and are only to be seen in couples. The keeper of a captive crane (*Grus grus*) induced it to dance by making the appropriate movements.

The arts of courtship, although not confined to birds, find their most elaborate development. among them.   To mention but a few other examples : the male uca has one claw much larger and more brilliantly coloured than the other, which is used for beckoning to the female.   Male antelopes engage in mimic battles, and male springbocks perform certain conventionalized movements in the presence of the females, springing about six feet into the air in a rigid posture and displaying their white manes.

Among the chimpanzees at Teneriffe, Rothmann and Teuber saw a male dancing in a triple rhythm close to a number of females ; and the sexual significance of its movements was obvious. One of the females also performed dancing movements in the presence of a male ; the resemblance between these dances and those of primitive races was very marked. Köhler watched his whole group of monkeys, playing, dancing, and leaping about without being able to detect any erotic element. These dances had not been learnt by imitation, and the animals welcomed to their dance their human owner whom they knew to be their friend.

How far dancing and the arts of courtship are traditional among animals or how far they must be regarded as purely instinctive is not yet known. It is, nevertheless, safe to assume that pure instinct preponderates (C > V). The presence of other animals is a necessary condition of the self-display in pairing dances and in the dances evolved from wooing movements. Here we find one of the fundamental reasons why human beings seek an audience for the display of their æsthetic activity (Gross). The peacock spreads the splendour of its tail whether the onlookers be swine or men (Darwin). Yet in singing birds the impulse to sing is so strong that it asserts itself even when they are alone. When singing, dancing, or flying games are performed in common, they may legitimately be described as forms of social self-display.

E PLAY

The cause of play is the impulse which drives every animal to be doing something ; the purpose of play, especially during youth, is often the acquisition of skill in some activity useful to the animal ; on the other hand, play may be an end in itself. In the case of some animals (young birds and mammals in particular) and children, this joy in activity is at first aimless ; but as the child or the animal grows older, under the guidance of parents or teachers the activity pursues more and more definite aims, and in various ways assumes biological significance. Not infrequently play becomes merely a preparation for the so-called struggle for existence. It practically vanishes at the age of sexual maturity and gives way to purposeful activities, and in the domain of sex, love games takes its place. It has in itself no sexual reference, but it may acquire this character. When full-grown, children and animals distinguish without any difficulty between jest and earnest ; while playing they are always conscious of acting a part ; a dog at play only pretends to bite. It is, however, well known that jest may pass through various intervening stages to earnest.

An attempt has been made to derive the artistic activities of human beings from their play ; but this is inadmissible. It is true that the artistic impulse of primitive man may originally have expressed itself in play, as it does at first in the case of children. But later, with the progress of distinctively " human " development, the impulse has expressed itself more and more as a law to itself, and has produced the phenomena now found among the various races of man. Whoever would regard art as a development of the play impulse, must also regard all technical knowledge and skill, and finally all vocational human activities as having the same source ; for each of these occurs somewhere and somehow in the activities of children at play. To derive the artistic impulse from the play impulse is to confuse the latter with the universal desire to be doing something and to fall a victim to that endeavour which, in its extreme forms, can only be called a mania for derivation, and which consists in the effort always to refer one phenomenon back to another.

When Köhler's young chimpanzees were handling objects their activities almost always came under the heading of play. If during an experiment a novel form of activity was demanded by some necessity or other, it was quite certain that the innovation would reappear very soon afterwards on some occasion when the animals were " playing ", i.e. in circumstances where it had no practical utility, but was merely the expression of enhanced vitality. On the other hand, among the many games in which the monkeys made use of objects, some could easily be diverted into useful channels, as for instance stick-jumping, or digging with the said sticks. How the use of a tool might, in certain cases, have its origin in a game, may be told in Köhler's own words : " I certainly do not wish to maintain that the chimpanzee one day takes its stick, and so to speak, says to itself—of course, it cannot talk—' There, now I will dig for roots.' But no observer can doubt that when it has been digging in play, and has by chance come across roots, it will go on digging for them because it had long used its hands for this purpose, and now has discovered a better method."

The most intelligent animal was usually the moving spirit in the invention of any new game, and although in their play Köhler's chimpanzees constantly adopted new crazes, they never imitated human activities. One of their favourite forms of activity was to prize off the covers of the drain

pits, using sticks as levers. The attraction did not lie in the
foul contents of the drains so much as in the possibility of
smashing something to pieces. According to Köhler, if a
chimpanzee is confronted with something destructible it will
not rest until the object cannot be further broken up, or is
not worth breaking into smaller pieces.

Ladling liquid with bits of straw, small sticks, and so on
was often undertaken in play, even when the animals had
free access to water while feeding. Another fashion was
catching ants on small sticks and straws. One particular
animal invented this game, and the others quickly followed
its example. A straw, or something of the kind, was held
across the path of the ants, and when covered with the
insects was drawn through the mouth. Köhler thinks that
the sporting interest more than equalled the appetite for
ants ; as long as this sport was in fashion the chimpanzees
were always to be seen crouching together over the
pathway of the ants, each animal with a straw of its own,
looking like a row of fishermen beside a river. For a time the
fashionable game was poking the fowls with sticks. The
fowls were either decoyed, or actually fed, with bread, and
then poked violently with a stick ; this game was sometimes
played by two chimpanzees together, one of which fed the
fowl while the other poked it.

The chimpanzees were very fond of fastening, in some way
or another, a variety of different objects to their bodies.
Nearly every day Köhler would see an animal going about
with a cord, a shred of stuff, or a twig upon its head or
shoulders. The animals would play, not only with the
objects but with each other, and it was plain that the

drapery in some way added to their pleasure. This primitive form of adornment was not intended to produce an effect on other animals ; its sole result was an increase of self-consciousness in the wearer (the sort of feeling aroused in human beings by the wearing of a scarf, a sabre, or a top hat).

In interpreting the above games it must be borne in mind (1) that the chimpanzees were still young, and (2) that they were divorced from their natural surroundings, and that foraging was no longer a necessity ; they were, so to speak, unemployed, and play was the only available outlet for their active impulses. It is probable that chimpanzees living in their native forests are much less given to playing.

Speaking generally, it is especially young animals which play together, but older animals do so too. Full-grown apes in their native forests romp together in a way that can only be described as a movement game. Not only members of the same species, but members of different species will play together, especially in captivity. Nevertheless, great care must always be taken to avoid any confusion between real hunting, pairing dances, etc., and genuine play. Play often contains an element of rivalry, e.g. in sham fighting and in hunting games.

We may follow Groos in distinguishing three types of the latter, those with living prey (cat and mouse), those with living mock prey (one dog pursuing another), and those with inanimate mock prey (ball games).

According to Pfungst, young wolves and dogs organize fighting games and hunting games with mock prey, which may be either alive or dead ; and during these games young wolves display the rudiments of retrieving, although they lack all previous training. According to Brehm a young orang outan clearly showed itself to be peculiarly attracted to small children, since it often tried to induce them to play with it by offering them its own playthings. When this orang utan saw itself unexpectedly in a mirror at first it took to its heels, and repeated this several times ; it then spat at its image and pelted it with all sorts of objects. In the end, however, it tried to induce its own image to play with it.

According to Schmidt, when kittens play it is partly at the instigation of the mother cat, and partly of their own accord ; the mother brings a half-dead mouse, or something of the kind, and the kittens then practise upon it. Among apes, on the contrary, according to Pfungst, games between a mother and child are always started by the latter ; the accounts of von Allersh seem, however, to indicate that among chimpanzees, in any case, the initiative is sometimes taken by the mother. Dogs, because they are more sociable, indulge in play to a greater extent than cats. Dogs, cats, apes, and other mammals play more often, and more whole-heartedly, with children than with adults, and put up with more from children ; they manifestly possess a certain understanding for the helplessness of childhood. If young mammals turn their play into earnest the mother not uncommonly separates the disputants.

Brehm describes a certain mode of behaviour found among chamois, which can only be described as play. When left completely undisturbed, chamois will squat on their haunches and slide, one after another, down slopes of snow

for a distance of a hundred to a hundred and fifty yards,
then climb back to the starting point, and begin the slide
all over again.

Schjelderup-Ebbe describes a kind of game, possessing a
certain sexual implication, found among wild duck, which are
monogamous. This author watched a mated female amuse
herself on several occasions by fooling unmated males;
she would fly towards them, but always retreated to safety
as soon as they began to pursue her.

It cannot be doubted that ants play at fighting; the fact
has been demonstrated by Huber, Forel, MacCook, Bates
(quoted from Groos, p. 147; Escherich, p. 188; Forel,
vol. iii, p. 88).

F   Uttering Sounds in Chorus

In the animal kingdom sounds are uttered in chorus, sometimes from pure imitation, sometimes as a group signal, and
sometimes without any definite motive. There is, further, the
alternating song of rival males, and the cry of greeting by
which excitement is expressed. These categories are often
not separated from one another by any sharp line of cleavage.

If a lion, either caged or free, begins to roar, any lions in
the neighbourhood immediately join in. A donkey braying
will set every other donkey within hearing braying, too.
Similarly a whole herd will bellow or howl when any one
animal gives the lead. Male frogs, inhabiting the same pond,
croak or are silent together, and even outside the pairing
season croak in chorus. The noise in the bird houses of a
zoological garden, where a bird is always prompted to

become vocal by the noises uttered by the rest, is known to everyone. Any noise may induce caged birds and tree frogs to sing or croak, while dogs begin to sing or howl when they hear music.

Wandering bands of animals emit call-notes continuously, e.g. the mixed bands of titmice, common creepers, wood-peckers, and golden-crested wrens. These group signals serve to keep the company together. Spring and autumn migrations are, on the contrary, carried out without calls ; it was a mistaken idea that the flocks are then kept together by such signals. When migrating, birds cry out only when bewildered or frightened, as, for instance, when they fly into the rays of a lighthouse, or over brightly lit cities, or when in daylight they catch sight of men. Like these titmice flocks, small groups of Marmosets traversing virgin forest continuously emit a thin piping or twittering sound Among *passalides*, or wood-boring beetles, mentioned several times already, where the two parents lead the family of larvæ, the members of the group give out a continuous chirping which keeps the band together.

Calling to each other in turn is a feature of the contests between male birds (e.g. among domestic cocks). The sounds emitted by *Tamias* are probably without any sexual meaning. About half a dozen each perched upon a stone, or other similar object, will chirp to one another hour after hour ; a distinct rhythm can sometimes be discerned in these sounds.

A pair of brooding cranes will send a cry of greeting to others of their own species passing in the air above ; two flocks of parrots will acknowledge each other with earsplitting shrieks. Two bats will call to one another if they chance to meet, and two swallows will do the same.

The sounds emitted by many kinds of apes form a genuine chorus. Thus a group of howling monkeys (*Alouetta*) do not set up a merely senseless howling, but really observe certain rules. The leading ape, an old male, acts as precentor (the Brazilians, on this account call him the " chaplain ") ; he begins with short staccato notes, and gradually lets his voice swell out into an organ peal. The remaining members of the band join in later with short phrases, but always limit themselves merely to the provision of an accompaniment. From time to time they all fall silent, then the leader begins again, and the concert proceeds as before. One and the same herd has sometimes been noticed to possess two choir leaders.

Among chimpanzees living in their natural surroundings an old male will begin intoning in a deep bass, and the whole troop will then join in ; the voices swell into a fortissimo and then gradually diminish until the concert dies away in the sounds emitted by one animal alone. This chanting takes place just after the animals wake, and while they are still in their nests ; it is also heard during the search for food, and especially on moonlight nights. *Colobus* monkeys sing in chorus during the day, particularly at dawn, in a manner peculiar to themselves ; the song begins softly and gradually attains considerable power ; if interrupted it is always taken up afresh shortly afterwards. South American sakis (*Pithecia*) come out of the forest morning and evening, collect in large herds and fill the air with penetrating cries. Gibbons and other species are also accustomed to emit hideous shrieks at sunrise and sunset. A characteristic feature of these choruses is that the apes always remain in the same spot while performing them.

G PROPERTY, PROVISIONS

Some animals at breeding time take possession of a particular domain, where they build their nests. Thus when pairing time begins each male stickleback lays claim to a special abode from which it drives away all other fishes. In an aquarium the boundaries of one male stickleback's domain are marked out from those of the rest only by fierce fighting. The females live meanwhile in swarms near the surface, and are fetched by the males to the nests each time they lay eggs.

In most bird species every pair lays exclusive claim at least to its own nest, and often to a certain radius round it as well. This domain may be either a bush, a piece of ground, a swamp, a small pond, or part of a stream ; the latter applies to moorhens (*Gallinula chloropus*), coots (*Fulica atra*), swans, and others. Thus the male wild duck drives every stranger of its own sex and species away from the brooding place ; in these struggles strange females may very likely be violated by force (von Geyr). When the pairing season is over the brooding place is, in many cases, abandoned, as happens among numerous species of thrushes, robins, dippers (*Cinclus*), different finches, cranes, swans, pond fowl, and water fowl. During the pairing season each male cuckoo occupies a sharply circumscribed domain ; the females rove from one male to another. One and the same male has been seen for decades in the same spot, and the females, too, return again and again to the same region. Every male nandu, with his harem, is master of a particular portion of land while the breeding season lasts. Although wild geese breed gregariously, each pair, nevertheless, claims as its own a certain area around its nest, and does not admit strangers within it. In a penguin colony each rectangle, bounded by pathways, belongs to the pair owning the nest built therein.

On the other hand, many birds of prey lay claim to the same domain throughout the year, that is to say beyond the brooding period, and suffer no rival within their boundaries. Thus every pair of eagles of the species *Haliaetus vocifer* rules a district about three kilometres in diameter. This is also true of other eagles, falcons, secretary birds, etc.

We also find the principle of territorial rights developed among some mammals. Every horde of apes possesses, as a rule, a clearly defined domain whose extent varies in different species. If two hordes encounter one another fierce fighting may ensue. Each herd of kangaroos possesses its own grazing place ; sometimes it possesses several, linked together by well-trodden paths. Herds of North American, prong-horned antelopes each inhabit a definite tract of country within which they travel long distances. In oriental cities every alley has its own half-wild dogs which do not dare to leave its shelter, since any dog entering a strange alley is attacked and torn to pieces by the dogs domiciled there.

Every ant-state has a special hunting ground, and if an ant belonging to one state trespasses on the territory of another a battle follows, the result of which is usually the

M

retreat of one of the parties ; it very seldom happens that two neighbouring states become used to and tolerate one another. On the other hand, the bee-states have property rights only within the hive ; the tracts of country where food is to be gathered are open to the members of any hive.

It is therefore no uncommon occurrence in the animal world for a single animal, a pair of animals, or a whole company to occupy either for a time, or permanently, a clearly defined domain. It happens less often that an animal looks upon some object as its own personal property. But some apes, for instance, will treat a plaything as their own. Brehm speaks of a captive baboon which took a tin can and other similar things with it to its sleeping place, and hid them there. A captive long-tailed monkey regarded as its own property, and used as playthings, rubber balls, corks, and bits of wood, etc. One or other of these objects was always for a time the most important (or, in other words, was the fashion), and was carried at night to the sleeping basket ; the others were carefully hidden behind and under cupboards, etc. The monkey regarded these objects as its own property and resented any attempt to touch them or take them away as an unjustifiable infringement of its rights. The animal was also in the habit of lodging smaller objects in its cheek pouches.

Some animals, both solitary and social, lay up stores of food over which they possess more or less clearly marked property rights. According to Schillings, when a leopard kills, after devouring the heart and the liver, and burying the entrails, it places the rest of its prey in storage among the branches of a tree or a bush, sometimes at a considerable height. The solitary and extremely unsocial hamster constructs one or more store chambers in its dwelling ; the mole, likewise a solitary creature, collects earthworms, and bites off their front ends to prevent them from escaping ; the squirrel, too, conceals provisions. Certain owls which always live alone bring back food and store it if their hunting has been particularly successful. A pair of shrikes (*Lanius*) usually store their prey (insects, amphibians, reptiles, small birds) on thorns all over their hunting ground.

Central American woodpeckers (*Melanerpe*) combine together to lay up stores for the winter, pecking holes in the bark of trees, and there hiding acorns. After the lapse of some weeks the whole flock returns and consumes the supply. Piping hares (*Ochotona*), which live together in colonies of burrows, collect great stores of hay, piling it up, and covering it during wet weather with broad-leaved plants. Alpine marmots live alone or in pairs in their summer nests, but in winter from five to fifteen of them inhabit the same nest, and these winter nests contain stores of hay.

How state-building insects collect and store food has already been described in detail. Male and female apothecary beetles (*Ateuchus sacer*), which live together in pairs within associations formed at some favourable place, make balls of dung and roll them hastily into holes previously prepared. During the process of conveying these balls to the burrows, their possession is fiercely disputed by other beetles. When the ball is safely housed, either the couple who made it devour it, or the female lays a single egg upon it, and the ball later serves to nourish the larva after it has been hatched.

IX GENERAL ANIMAL SOCIOLOGY (*continued*)

H Mutual Understanding and Imitation

As long as men alone are under consideration imitation and mutual understanding are two conceptions which seem to have little connexion with one another. But when we turn to the animal world we see that means of communication often merely lead animals to imitate some action performed by another. Behaviour of this kind lies midway between pure imitation, which is always spontaneous, and mutual comprehension of a higher order.

Pure imitation plays a great part among social animals. If one animal gives out its cry the rest usually follow suit ; such activities as running, flying into the air, consuming food, basking in the sun, etc., are all contagious. It is well known that the social instincts of some birds play tricks with them, and that hunters may lure them to destruction with the help of a decoy bird. If a young bird in the nest stirs its wings the rest of the brood immediately does the same. When penguins are hesitating at the edge of the ice, if one bird takes to the water all the rest follow its example. Zebras are very difficult to tame, and are taught their circus tricks by being given trained ponies as " instructors ". Captive gnus can be induced to make their peculiar capers if their keeper will jump into the air in front of them, and cranes will dance if appropriate movements are made before them.

The force of example is familiar to us from our acquaintance with our fellow creatures ; the infectious nature of yawning, eating, etc., is almost proverbial. In theatres and at concerts the audience lets itself be carried away over and over again by the persistent applause of one or a few. Talking is also infectious, and it is impossible to deny that human conversation rests upon the same instinctive basis as the social sounds produced by animals. For it is frequently practised, not with the object of imparting conversation, but for its own sake, as an expression of sociability.

Köhler could make every chimpanzee in the station look in exactly the same direction by suddenly behaving as though he were extremely frightened, and riveting a spell-bound gaze on a particular spot. All the chimpanzees would then run together as though thunderstruck, and stare at the same spot, even though nothing whatever was to be seen there. It is common knowledge that anybody can make the same experiment at any time with his fellow men by staring fixedly at a portion of the pavement, or into the air.

Apes possess, in a high measure, a propensity for imitation. According to Rothmann and Teuber, the Teneriffe chimpanzees learnt by watching alone to open doors, to insert a key in a lock, and to regulate the flow of a water supply by a valve. The chimpanzees tried to scrub the floor boards as they had seen their keeper do, and played leap-frog after watching some children at the game. According to von Oertzen, tame chimpanzees imitated the bodily movements of dancing negro women ; they also took an interest in the cowrie shell games of the natives, without,

of course, any understanding of the rules, cleaned their
teeth as the natives did, etc. ; and all this came about not
as a result of training, but from observation alone. Nevertheless it is unspeakably difficult for the chimpanzee to imitate
anything which it cannot in some measure understand. In
common with all other animals, it can imitate only those
actions which are included among its own entirely
spontaneous activities ; completely unintelligent imitation
never takes place. Chimpanzees and monkeys in general
which have been trained by showmen to perform special
tricks because they are so teachable, lead an empty, pseudo-
human life, and it is useless to argue from their behaviour
to the psychological states of other animals.

The peculiar manifestations of the mass mind are due to
imitation and the reciprocal stimulation of excitement.
Not only are swarms of locusts, dragon flies, etc., brought
into existence by these forces, but by them they are held
together, and impelled to uniform movements of flight.
Reciprocal imitation is responsible for changes of movement
and other joint actions in a herd, or any other group of
animals.

It has often been noticed that if a trained wild animal
suddenly falls upon its tamer, the rest of the performing
animals in the cage join in the attack. According to
Sokolowsky, this common action is instigated, not by some
mysterious understanding between the animals, but by
observation of the movements of the animal which begins
the attack. In the same way many of the animals which
live in herds imitate each other's movements in taking to
flight or attacking, although the majority may remain

unaware of the necessity of the action which prompted the action they are copying. A horse reacts very markedly to the noise of another horse galloping. Frogs living in associations are put on the alert by the noise made by one of their companions taking to the water (the splash sound, Yerkes). Many animals develop a characteristic note of warning; birds utter a special kind of cry; chamois and marmots whistle; the wild rabbit beats the earth with its hind legs, and kangaroos sound an alarm in the same way. Animals, whether social or solitary, often understand immediately a cry of fear or a cry of warning uttered by another species; one species of bird will take heed of the warning cries of another and mammals take warning from birds. Goats and fowls understand each other's danger signals (Schmid). On hearing the warning whistle of the reedbuck (*Redunca*), not only members of the same species, but waterbucks (*Kobus*), ibis, and herons all take to flight. In East Africa the spurred peewit warns all the animals of the plain of the arrival of a newcomer with its cry, which it utters as it flies from place to place.

Many animals also draw the appropriate conclusion from the flight of others belonging to quite different species.

Cattle heron perch on the backs of wild buffalo and elephants, ox-peckers (*Buphaya*) on rhinoceros, cattle, elephants, buffaloes, antelopes, and giraffes, the dotterel (*Pluvianus*) on crocodiles, the ox-bird (*Textor albirostris*) on buffaloes. These birds search the hides of their hosts for parasites, and warn the great beasts of the presence of intruders by flying away, and sometimes by cries as well. This warning is not, of course, given intentionally. The

process is reversed when hunters are guided to the resting
places and travel routes of wild animals, especially those of
elephants and buffaloes, by watching the movements of the
cattle heron (Berger). When the ox-pecker keeps company
with tame cattle it shows no fear of men ; but when it
allies itself with wild animals it is extraordinarily shy and
circumspect, thus adapting its behaviour to the example set
by the particular mammal whose society it has adopted.

The honey-guide (*Indicator*), a bird, cries out whenever
it sees a man or a ratel (*Mellivora*) ; if the newcomer will
follow, it flies ahead in stages, and leads the way to a nest
of wild bees. If, then, the man or the badger robs the nest,
the honey-guide profits by eating the bee-brood. It is
probable that originally the instinct was bound up with
badgers only ; later the birds came to know that men, too,
rob bee-hives, so that now, as a result of habit and tradition,
they also set up their crying whenever they see a man. A
further instance of symbiosis, where the movements of
one species are guided by those of another, is furnished by
sharks and their pilot-fishes. The pilot-fish guides the shark
to any prey which it may have sighted, but does not itself
attack the spoil, though it perhaps eats any stray morsel
that comes its way. When in the company of a single shark
the pilot-fish is well protected from enemies ; when several
sharks swim together pilot-fishes are absent. Led by their
following instinct, these fishes will accompany sailing boats,
floating pieces of wood, casks, etc.

One animal will often use another as a guide in discovering
sources of food. If ravens see a member of their own species
dart downwards in a straight line they make for the same

spot ; this is also true of vultures, who sometimes, too, come
to earth if they see a mass of ravens on the ground, since it
is only on carrion that ravens crowd close together. Jackals
will hasten at full gallop to the place where a vulture has
alighted, expecting to find prey there (Berger, p. 125).
According to Schillings, vultures in Africa sometimes guide
the natives involuntarily to a place where a lion has made a
kill, thus procuring them a meal. Gulls, too, follow one
another, and also in the wake of ships, since experience has
taught them that food is constantly to be found there.
Frigate birds keep watch on dolphins and other fishes of
prey, and when these drive a swarm of flying fishes
above the surface of the water the frigate birds pounce upon
the latter. Dragon flies keep pace exactly with horses,
circling round them, not because they are particularly
attached to these animals, but on account of the flies to
be caught in their neighbourhood.

The call notes which some birds produce unceasingly, as
well as those emitted by monkeys and beetles, have already
been mentioned and recognized as a means of mutual
understanding and as flock signals which serve to hold a
company together. Tame cattle, similarly, pay heed to an
artificial guiding sound, the bell belonging to their own
herd. Among some of the mammals which live in herds a
special smell belonging to the secretions of certain glands
is the sign which keeps the herd together. In some species
of birds white spots and stripes, visible perhaps only during
flight, are the marks of identity by means of which
two members of the same species recognize one another,
just as among men signs of rank or numbers serve as

distinguishing marks upon uniforms, etc. In the same way the white patch which adorns the rump of many kinds of deer is regarded as an identification mark which enables an animal to follow its leader and its herd. The patch is conspicuous on roe-deer only during the winter ; this is said to be connected with the fact that in summer the females live alone with their young. When Japanese deer (*Pseudaxis sica*) are at rest, no patch is visible, but it becomes broad and clear when they take to flight.

According to Berger, wild animals without this white patch generally have tails strikingly light in colour on the underside, and their habit of wagging their tails when in flight is their method of displaying this guiding mark. According to Schillings, giraffes always lash their tails powerfully when in flight, or if their suspicions are aroused. He certainly goes too far when he asserts that although giraffes are completely dumb, these movements of their tails are " signals " by means of which they " convey their thoughts to one another " ; it is, however, perfectly imaginable that an animal whose suspicions have been aroused will set its companions on the alert by lashing its tail.

Among the higher vertebrates (birds and mammals) expressive movements are largely used as a means of mutual intelligence between one animal and another, and it is probably fair to suppose that such means take their origin, phylogenetically, in expressive sounds and movements.

According to Köhler, Pfungst, Brehm, and every competent authority, there is no species of ape in which the expression of emotion attains to the rank of an " ape-

language ", as Garner erroneously imagined ; even among
chimpanzees, according to Köhler, no communication is
ever made through any phonetic or other designation of
objects. The alleged ape-language discovered by Garner
was composed only of sounds expressing pleasure or dis-
pleasure ; it is for this reason that it is possible to make an
ape take promptly to its heels by reproducing a cry of fear
on the gramophone ; or, by reproducing a cry of hunger,
to induce a corresponding state of excitement in the animal.
According to Brehm the forms of expression in use among
apes fall into distinct and different groups, which differ even
among different species of the same genus ; when members of
these different species encounter one another in the common
cage of a zoological garden, at first they either entirely fail
to understand one another, or else, as very frequently
happens, misunderstand one another to the point of open
hostility. Only gradually do the different species make
friends with their fellow-prisoners, and learn to interpret
the sounds made by them. Each newcomer must first bite
its way into a recognized position ; this, according to Brehm,
is a long-established phenomenon among captive animals,
the result being that an exactly ordered social scale comes
into existence, in which every individual has a perfectly
definite rank (compare here Schjelderup-Ebbes' experiments
in connexion with the " pecking-order " of a flock of fowls).
Every ape species and every group of nearly related species
has its own special noises, lip-signs, bodily deportment, and
movements which it uses for intercourse. It would be of the
greatest possible interest to establish how far these methods
of communication are traditional, and how far they are based

upon instinct (using human beings as a comparison : a newly born infant sucks quite instinctively without any guidance ; the first attempts at speech are instinctive, but the traditions of the environment determine which language it learns). In the Berlin Zoological Gardens the way in which the apes conduct themselves towards each other has been designated for years as the " ape-code ".

Pfungst declares that there was no authenticated case of weeping among the apes under his observation (compare against this what Rothmann and Teuber have to say of chimpanzees). Vocal expressions are richest and most numerous among the apes of the New World, and this is correlated with a certain poverty of gesture. Some of the motor manifestations agree in meaning and expression with those of men, e.g. the grinning of drills and mandrills ; Pfungst interprets this grinning as a playful display of their weapons, the eye-teeth, which occurs as they lift the corners of the mouth as a sign of goodwill ;   and he comes to the conclusion that our assertion should not be of the form that " apes laugh, too ", but that " men laugh, too, although they no longer bite ". It seems to me, nevertheless, very doubtful whether the display of the eye-teeth (which are used as weapons), is the most important factor in the phylogenetic origin of laughter ; on the contrary, I believe that the eye-teeth in their quality of weapons played absolutely no part in originating laughter. Some gestures are identical in appearance with those of men, but possess an entirely different meaning ; thus, for instance, nodding the head is a sign of anger in baboons.

Since most of the gestures made by apes are completely

unlike those made by men, they have often been misinterpreted. No trace is to be found of that " sénse of the comic " so frequently assigned to them. Grinding the teeth, chewing movements of the jaws, or opening the mouth widely all serve to display an ever-ready weapon, and thus denote rage. Baring clenched teeth, which being clenched are not prepared for fighting, is a sign of fear in many species. Pfungst believes that smacking the lips, with simultaneous movements of the tongue, originally expressed the foretaste of some toothsome morsel, and afterwards came to be a friendly gesture of greeting ; it is also used to manifest a willingness to search through the coat of a companion, which, among apes, is an eagerly desired attention. In the course of this process, usually described as " louse-hunting ", scurf, scraps of dirt, etc., are eaten, but not vermin, from which the animals, in captivity at least, are nearly always free.

Presenting the hindquarters is not, as has been imagined, either a threat, a sign of contempt, nor a defensive action, and even in the females it is not generally an invitation to copulate, but rather a mark of submissive friendliness and humility ; the gesture is performed by young as well as by full-grown animals of both sexes, and they perform it before their own images in a mirror in just the same way. This greeting is only offered to their keepers in early days, and is abandoned as time goes on, possibly because the relation of dependence between them is fixed once for all, and perfectly well understood by both parties (Brehm). It would be of the greatest interest to establish how much of this ceremony, the " ape-greeting ", is learnt, and how much is purely instinctive.

According to Rothmann and Teuber, the chimpanzee has at command an extraordinary variety of facial expression which includes that of mute laughter, weeping (without tears! but compare Köhler), joy, fear, rage, all the different grades of desire, disillusionment, jealousy, etc. This opens up the possibility of extensive communication between the animals. Expressive gestures of the arms are also highly developed among chimpanzees. Holding out the arms when the body is bowed and prone expresses a desire for pity or forgiveness. Ducking and presenting the hindquarters frequently signifies friendly submission ; according to Rothmann and Teuber, the sexual origin of this gesture is often apparent. The animals were repeatedly noticed to touch each other with their mouths, kissing fashion ; this always meant that a piece of chewed fruit was being passed from one animal's mouth into the mouth of a friend. The origin of human kisses most probably lies in this custom ; among human beings, too, the passing of morsels of food from lip to lip is a form of erotic expression.

According to Pfungst wolves have ten different tones at their disposal ; half of these are expressive of anger ; if they are actually menaced, even young wolves kept in complete isolation set up a genuine baying. The view that they learn to do this by copying dogs, or that the baying is an imitation of the human voice, is thus rendered untenable. The domestic dog obviously barks more frequently because it is free from the restraints which force a wild animal to keep silence ; thus barking, originally a method of expressing anger, becomes adapted to the utterance of other emotions, e.g. joy. Young male wolves have a habit of spontaneously presenting the paw, which is expressive of a wish to make friendly advances. To show itself defenceless, a wolf rolls on to its back. To urinate frequently is a method of social intercourse. Among wolves and dogs scratching after defeacating is, according to Darwin, prompted by a rudiment of the instinct to cover over excrement ; but Pfungst believes it due rather to an instinct to disseminate its own scent. The fact that some animals deposit their excrement on raised places, e.g. on stones, is held to support this view.

Under natural conditions, hamsters, badgers, martins, and rabbits void their excrement in special places. All species of lamas, and different species of antelopes, form heaps of excrement ; and, in the case of guanos, when one of the heaps reaches a certain size another is begun near it. Hartebeests deposit their dung on a special circular area, trodden flat, in the middle of which stands a small ant-heap covered by stale dung. The levelling is brought about by a herd collecting on and near an ant-hill, turning the spot into a romping ground and trampling it flat. Berger has an illustration (p. 24) of one such deposit made by hartebeests. Schillings declares that the African rhinoceros (*Rhinoceros bicornis*) takes special pains to drop its dung in definite places, afterwards scattering it by scraping the ground with its hind legs. Schillings believes that the dung heaps serve as posts and guiding points by means of which the widely scattered animals can gather together again. A similar purpose is attributed to the action of the hippopotamus, which habitually scatters its dung over bushes with the help of its brush-like tail, covered with short stiff bristles.

A brief discussion of those animals which are supposed to communicate information by taps on the ground may be introduced at this point. It is not possible to take the accounts at present available into serious consideration, since, though very circumstantial, they are also quite uncritical. According to Guenther, something of great importance has never yet been seen to take place ; appropriate action has not been observed to follow a communication grasped by the intellect. If one of these talking dogs is told " there is a cake for you in the next room. Go and fetch it," it does not do as it is commanded, but taps out some answer or other, its behaviour being thus directly contrary to that which dogs, as a rule, exhibit. Guenther's objection is certainly well worth consideration, but it is, nevertheless, always possible to object that here, once more, we may be faced by one of those riddles with which the mentality of men and of animals so often confront us.

Ants communicate by means of their "antennal language" (Escherich, p. 303, Eidmann). This " language " is no more than certain contacts of the antennæ serving to support the social instincts by communicating to one ant the emotions of another. Ants greatly desire this mutual contact through the antennæ, and if the need is left unsatisfied for any length of time they become deeply disturbed. It is used to excite the imitative instinct, as a summons to partake of food or to change the nest, to indicate that by following the guide food may be reached, to incite to attack or to flight, to give warning of danger, and to soothe excited companions ; antennal taps are also used to indicate the path of a migration. The signs conveyed differ according to the strength of the taps, their frequency and their location. Probably the odorous particles adhering to the antennæ (for prey, etc.) also play a certain part in communicating information. An ant lays emphasis on some communications by pushing its head against the breast of its companion. In a summons to food, the forelegs are made use of in addition to the antennæ, and the companion is licked in the region of the mouth. If warning alone has no effect, force is used to drag companions away from danger.

It has been noticed that when an ant discovers prey it taps another, and the latter betakes itself unaccompanied to the spoil, while the former departs to fetch further assistance. An alarm is rapidly spread from ant to ant throughout the nest by means of taps of the antennæ. Soldier ants also spread warning by knocking, or by special chirping noises. It has already been described how some guests of the ants are in a high degree adapted to life in an ant's nest. In this connexion it is worthy of especial note that the *Claviger* and *Lomechusa* beetles use their antennæ for tapping the ants just as the ants are accustomed to do in their communications with each other. These beetles touch the ants they encounter with their antennæ, cross them with those of the ants, tap the backs and sides of the latter, and stroke their cheeks if they want food.

Unfortunately we know much less about means of communication among termites than among ants; but the organized activity of the members of a termite state is a sure sign that termites also must have brought their methods of communication to a very high degree of development.

Among honey bees certain of the notes which they utter

have an extremely contagious effect, and result in the performance of some united action. Thus the characteristic swarming note issuing from one hive may induce another hive to swarm, although the time may not be ripe for it to do so. The stinging note given out by one bee will urge others to the attack, and the sting odour, i.e. the odour of the poison injected, has here a contributing effect. A queenless hive lifts up the mourning cry, and there are many other tones, e.g. the note of hunger, which inform an experienced bee-keeper of the state of affairs in the hive at any given moment.

Von Frisch has shown how honey bees communicate information to one another whilst engaged in the search for food. If a bee finds a particularly plentiful source of honey, on each return to the hive it executes a kind of round dance on the honey-comb ; this throws the bees clustering near it into a state of great excitement, and induces many of them to fly out in search of the source of the supply. If their loads are small, the homing bees refrain from dancing, and in this case their neighbours remain in the hive. Thus dancing is a method of informing the hive that a remunerative load is somewhere awaiting them. It is erroneous to suppose that a bee which has found a source of food escorts other members of the hive to the same locality. On the contrary the bees which fly out after the dance depart quite independently of the dancer, and search the country in all directions for the particular flower scent which clung to the dancing bee. This scent they have impressed on their memory by following the dancer about the hive and exploring the hinder part of its body with their organs of smell, the antennæ.

Another organ of communication is brought into use, especially in connexion with odourless sources of food. This is a pouch rich in glands, which, when it is extruded, gives out an odour perceptible even to men. The workers engaged in exploiting a rich source of supply, on arriving at their goal from the hive, circle round the former for some time with this organ extruded ; it is kept in this position while they suck the honey, and in this way the neighbourhood is impregnated with the peculiar odour which emanates from the organ. This serves to attract the newcomers from the hive as they fly hither and thither in search of the spot. The special sound given out by the wings of workers frequenting a rich source of supply plays no part in attracting new-comers. If, owing to weather conditions, the productive crop of nectar temporarily runs dry, the workers revisit the spot from time to time to inspect the process of its renewal.

The pollen gatherers communicate the whereabouts of a locality rich in pollen to one another, just as the nectar gatherers of the hive do in the case of nectar, by means of a dance. This dance, however, is a sort of " tail dance " rather than a " round dance ", and in this case the special scent of the pollen brought in serves as a guide to the flowers from which it is obtained.

I   Pure Instinct, Habit, Tradition

Many of the actions which in the case of human beings are determined by tradition $(C < V)$, are regulated among animals by pure instinct $(C > V)$; it is, nevertheless, necessary to point out that where animals are concerned we are far from being able to declare in every case how much depends upon tradition, and how much upon pure instinct. In human beings tradition has to make good the comparative lack of instinctive certainty; hence the multiplicity of customs and opinions found among related and neighbouring tribes, and even among the different professions and classes of a single nation. The flexibility of human behaviour and the possibility of progress in the sense of an increase of knowledge are both dependent upon the fact that the majority of men's actions have to be learnt and practised, while a minority only are determined once and for all by instinct. Were it possible that among ants or spiders, as among men, some were learned (the reason this cannot be is that $C > V$), it is certain that these learned individuals would look upon themselves and the members of their own race as the key-stone of creation, assigning to men a comparatively low place in the order of creation on account of the very small number of specialized instincts possessed by them; for the criterion of high spiritual qualities, and the place to be assigned to those possessing them in a duly constituted society would naturally be, from the point of view of ants or spiders, the possession of instincts as highly specialized as possible.

The solitary spider builds its ingenious nest without pattern and without guidance; the process is, therefore, purely " intuitive ". Among state-building instincts it is the unfailing certainty (so hard for us to imagine) of the instincts implanted in each individual which guarantees the continued existence of the community as a whole. But observations recently published by Wasmann and Rüschkamp indicate that among ants (in addition to instinct) tradition and example may also play a part in fashioning behaviour. Wasmann showed that in a mixed colony workers of a certain species normally living underground behaved like the members of the species associated with them, and would go forth with them into bright sunshine to visit the leaf and scale insects. The innate instinct, in this case, was obviously modified on the one hand by direct imitation of the behaviour of companions, and on the other by means of the "antennæ language" with the help of which ants incite their companions of the same colony to share their own activities. Rüschkamp found the same sort of thing in the mixed colony under his observation; he further noticed that one of the two associated species infected by the example of the other not only took to rearing root-eating aphides instead of bark-eating aphides but even went so far as to make a complete change in their method of nest-building. The facts here related are of the greatest interest from the point of view of animal psychology, and it is very much to be hoped that ant investigators will in future also pay particular attention to any possible modifications of instinct.

It has already been shown that for young birds and mammals the instruction of their parents, or, at the least, the example set by them and by other members of the community, may be of great importance. Among those fishes, too, which tend their brood, the example of the parents may perhaps influence the manner of seeking for prey and avoiding danger. The fear of man is traditional and not purely instinctive in animals; for all travellers who penetrate to regions hitherto unexplored by man are unanimous in describing the animals inhabiting these

districts as altogether unafraid ; it is only gradually that
they learn to flee their worst enemy, and the knowledge is
handed down from generation to generation through the
example of the older animals. According to Morgan, during
the two years which followed the first erection of telegraph
wires in Scotland, numberless white grouse flew into them
and were destroyed ; later they learned, through tradition,
to shun the danger. According to this author, too, the fear
shown by birds and mammals at the sight of certain enemies
is the result of experience and tradition. This fear is com-
municated by cries of warning which are themselves
instinctive ; but the understanding of these cries is the result
of experience and tradition.   At first young birds and
mammals instinctively react to any large object moving
quickly ; with the growth of experience it is only the
unaccustomed which evokes the reaction of fear. Cries of
warning are likewise understood by animals of other species ;
and these cries are also uttered by animals which have not
themselves caught sight of the enemy, but have only heard
the first alarm. Just as it is a tradition among some species
to fly from men, others again seek their company ; it is
through tradition that swallows and white storks have
become the household companions of men, and nest only on
human dwellings.

According to Morgan, newly hatched ostriches and Assam
pheasants die of hunger if the breeder does not direct their
attention to food by means of pecking movements. In the
case of young pheasants belonging to other species, however,
and young chickens, scratching and pecking is purely
instinctive. Experience teaches them that to scratch among

loose earth is profitable, while scratching on hard ground is unprofitable ; and in a short time the chicks learn to distinguish in their pecking between edible and inedible objects. But it is always easier to rear young birds when they have old birds to imitate in eating and drinking, etc. Chicks in many instances also imitate each other. A breeder can teach young pigeons, separated from their parents, to pick up grain by putting them among young fowls, whose pecking they quickly imitate. A hen teaches her chicks to peck by taking up objects and letting them fall before their eyes. But even though a chicken will develop into an ordinary fowl without imitating the mother bird, its instinctive activities come into play earlier and with greater certainty when it has the opportunity of doing so. The same is true of other birds ; a bird will learn to fly without being taught by its parents, merely taking longer than it would otherwise do. In the case of ants, Heyde has established that if young ants are separated from their elders every activity, particularly nest-building and fighting, manifests itself later than is customary. Thus normally the actions of older animals incite imitation in those which are younger.

Coming into contact with members of their own species is an event of great importance for young dogs kept in isolation from birth ; they then come under the influence of traditional canine behaviour. Young beasts of prey reared in isolation would doubtless develop predatory methods similar to those of animals which had enjoyed the advantage of parental instruction ; but theirs would probably be found to lack polish. Tradition is of great importance to all those animals which live in herds. The individual, in these cases, is born into a group of animals accustomed to perform a number of actions after a special fashion. With the help of the instinct of imitation it makes these ways and methods its own, and tradition hands these on from generation to generation. The dams built by Canadian and European beavers are said to be hundreds and thousands of years old ; thus countless generations have worked at them and taken pains to preserve them. In more densely populated countries, however, the beaver now usually inhabits simple subterranean burrows, and no longer builds itself a fort.

It may also be through tradition that the solitary honey-guide (*Indicator*) has acquired the habit of crying out not only when it sees a ratel but also when it sees a man. The Egyptian kite (*Milvus ægyptius*) makes an exact study of the habits of the human beings in its neighbourhood and awaits just the right moment in which to snatch its plunder. It attempts to profit in the same way from the hunting of other birds of prey, and follows hunters in the expectation of booty.

Young water birds swim purely instinctively and quite perfectly as soon as they emerge from the egg ; the American squirrel, captured in infancy and separated from its parents will hide away nuts in a room just as a wild squirrel hides them in a hollow tree, performing all the movements necessary for this action in the manner characteristic of the species. Wallace and others believed that birds build their nests solely by tradition and imitation. Nevertheless, it has been proved that birds which have never watched the building of a nest, nor inhabited one in their youth, will yet build after the manner of their species. It is, however, true that old birds build more perfectly than young ones, so that practice is certainly of importance. In just the same way older harvest mice build their nests more skilfully than their younger companions.

It is debatable whether the nest-building habits of anthropoid apes are traditional or purely instinctive. Köhler believes the latter to be the case. And Brehm is of the same opinion concerning orangs. But it must be remembered that Köhler's chimpanzees were at least five years old when they reached Tenerife ; thus they may very well have learnt to build nests beforehand in their free state or may at least have watched the process. According to Reichenow the nest-building instinct only makes its appearance in gorillas when these animals have lived under natural conditions up to a certain age, and not when they have been captured in infancy. It is, in addition, largely unknown how much of the behaviour of anthropoid apes should be regarded as traditional, and how much as purely instinctive. Consequently we are also ignorant whether, so far as their habits of life and expressive movements, etc., are concerned, differences are to be found between the different breeds of chimpanzees and other species, similar to those often found between nearly related and closely neighbouring races of men.

One of the most obscure riddles of animal psychology is the yearly migration of birds. Attempts have been made to prove that knowledge of the migrating routes is traditional. But this could only hold good for those species in which young and old travel together, e.g. swallows and storks. The explanation is worthless when applied to species whose members are divided into classes according to their age, and in which the younger birds set out a few weeks before the older ones, e.g. starlings and crows. Ornithologists do not believe that the single older birds which take to flight at the same time as the younger ones serve as guides to the latter. Tradition seems to be altogether ruled out in the case of the species whose members, including the young birds, migrate alone, e.g. many birds of prey, certain species of singing birds, cuckoos, and hoopoes. The fact that even when birds are taken very young from the nest they are attacked by great restlessness at the migrating season seems to indicate that migration is instinctive. Experiments made with the help of rings have shown that certain individual birds, at least, return year after year to the same winter quarters, following always exactly the same route on their journey (Baldwin).

Cranes, herons, geese, ducks, swans, flamingoes, snipe, dotterels, all fly in V-formation ; one side of the V is usually longer than the other. If the flock is large a W is formed ; if it is small the birds often fly in a single slanting line. Young geese, still unable to fly, also form such a slanting graded line when swimming in the wake of their parents. The adoption of the arrow-head formation in flying is not traditional but purely instinctive, for it is characteristic of young wild geese which have been hatched out in captivity by domestic hens. The biological significance of the arrow-head formation is that for certain ærodynamic reasons it lightens the labour of flying for each individual bird ; the term " resonance flight " (Resonanzflug) is used in this connexion. The leader, who has the heaviest work to do, is frequently relieved ; the long side of the V is, as a rule,

turned in the direction from which the wind is blowing;
ibis, curlews and oyster-catchers fly in a long line, side by
side; starlings in large swarms with a wide front; storks,
larks, finches, yellow-hammers, thrushes, swallows and
swifts in irregular flocks. The hooded crow flies in open
formation, one bird after another.

In the songs of birds it is necessary to distinguish between
inherited and acquired factors (Naumann, Haecker and
others). The distinctive character of the notes emitted
(fluting, whistling, twittering, power of modulation, rhythm)
belongs to the innate endowment of each young bird and
depends upon the structure of the vocal organs and inherited
brain capacity. This inborn, purely instinctive song, however, is perfected, in each individual case, by instruction;
and this, in the young birds of any given species, depends
entirely upon example, whether the example be that of the
parent bird or of an unrelated stranger. This explains the
well-known fact that chaffinches sing much worse in some
districts than in others not far distant. Here, then, tradition
plays an important part. It is a familiar fact to breeders
of chaffinches and canaries that a good singer trains good
pupils, but that good pupils are ruined by a bad singer.
This is also true of nightingales. In districts where they are
protected against marauders, of whatever kind, there are,
naturally, many very old birds whose songs grow better
and purer and stronger from year to year, and who thus
provide instruction of progressive excellence for the young
birds. In such districts the song of the nightingales undergoes a gradual improvement, whereas in places where the
birds do not live to any great age the singing gradually

deteriorates (Naumann). If a young male nightingale is procured in autumn from a second brood it may be a source of the greatest disappointment, for it will never have heard an old male singing, and will be unable to sing well without this guidance.

The relation between the morphological structure of the vocal organs, the instinct to sing, and individual acquirements, is most clearly displayed in the case of the so-called mocking birds, which weave into their natural song the notes of other birds as well as other sounds. Young birds brought up by foster parents belonging to another species may sometimes adopt the song of the latter. It is possible to train some birds (ravens, bullfinches, parrots) to repeat the sounds of human speech. The fact that birds belonging to the most dissimilar species are found in both these lists, is, according to Haecker, primarily an indication that the not inconsiderable variations in the vocal organs are of less importance to singing power than differences of mental endowment. Haecker maintains that the cases in which the female bird possesses a melodious song (canaries, robins, larks, bullfinches) can be fairly easily explained ; for, on the one hand, the female possesses, like the male, the necessary anatomical basis of song, and on the other, even the male has to acquire his real melody by a process of learning. Among birds, therefore, it is the varying development of mental capacity, and in particular of the instinct to sing, which lies at the root of the difference between the song of the male and the song of the female. The young of all, except mocking birds, instinctively choose one of their own species as a model. It therefore becomes clear that the necessary presupposition of imitation is an instinctive, intuitive, primary, and consequently not acquired knowledge of the ideal best suited to the peculiar nature of each bird.

Young birds, accustomed from their earliest moments to the sight of their keeper, cling to him and follow him ; and it is afterwards difficult, if not impossible, to induce them to attach themselves to their parents. This is also true of mammals. Among sheep it is through experience alone that a lamb learns to recognize his own dam; it is even possible for a lamb to fly in terror from its mother and follow almost any other large living creature. In order to overcome the mutual dislike of horses and donkeys, mule-breeders place young donkey foals, soon after their birth, with brood mares. In this way the donkey may become so completely accustomed to horses that when full-grown it cannot, by any means, be induced to pair with a female of its own species, and will only cover mares (Brehm, iii ; Aufl., vol. iii, p. 76). Thus, here, as in certain other instances, the " call of the blood " apparently fails to make itself heard. According to Whitman, if a pigeon is brought up by parents of another species it associates and pairs only with members of its adopted, and not with those of its own, race.

It is thus habit, and not an instinctive recognition of breed or species, which is the deciding factor (compare the national consciousness exhibited by human beings which has no necessary connexion with race). Among parrots kept in captivity love-making sometimes occurs between two birds of different species and the ties formed are not dissolved even if later one of the partners has the chance of pairing with a member of its own species.

Even parental instinct may be modified by habit. Morgan describes the behaviour of hens which have hatched out three successive broods of ducklings and thereby become accustomed to seeing the latter take to the water. When on the next occasion these hens were given hens' eggs to hatch out they made the most pressing attempts to induce the young chicks to take to the water, and even went so far as to push them in. It may here be pointed out that a hen which has already reared several broods of chickens is very much more disturbed when ducklings which she has hatched out make for water than a hen whose first brood behaves in this way.

J   DOMESTICATION

Needless to say, a breeder cannot produce something entirely new ; he can only select from within the range of possible variations provided by his animals, and by breeding bring the desired quality to greater perfection. Through methodical crossing he may unite valuable characteristics in one stock ; he is further able so to improve the living conditions of his domesticated animals that the desired characteristics can attain their fullest development. Some tame animals have undergone such changes in the course of their domestication that if set free they would succumb ; others when freed regain the physique and mentality of their natural state, i.e. they become wild again. (Krieg has written papers which are well worth reading on the return to the savage state among men and animals as he has himself observed it in South America.)

The animals which man has domesticated are, chiefly, members of social species ; for animals living in herds are far more easily and completely tamed than those which lead a solitary life. Not every social species, however, lends itself to domestication. Man keeps tame animals because he is himself a social being. The tame animal and its keeper together form an organized society in which the man is the master, the animal the inferior (in Schjelderup-Ebbe's sense). The question of superiority is settled once for all. In this case the organized society holds together because the instinct of subordination in the inferior is correlated with the ruling instinct of the master. It is not utility alone which leads men to keep tame animals ; there is in addition the irrational element of his desire to command and to protect. Here, again, the social bond is stronger than the bond of race or species ; the dog protects its master against other dogs and is incited by him to attack other men.

According to Brehm, South American Indian women suckle apes, opossums and agoutis, along with their own children, and display the same tenderness of look and bearing for these animals. For it is the chief pride of these women to possess a large number of tame domesticated animals. Any young mammal they can capture they take to their own breasts and this leads to such affection on the part of these animals, of the apes in particular, that they follow her wherever she goes. All love for animals arises from a fostering instinct difficult to account for on purely rational grounds, and the animals concerned attach themselves with varying degrees of affection to their protectors from their natural desire for companionship ; they behave well or badly according to the treatment meted out to them. Apes can sometimes be incited by their masters to attack men, fowls and other animals ; and, like dogs, they defend their masters. Jealousy is an emotion by no means unknown to many animals under human care ; a tame animal often greets its master with lively movements of its body and loud cries. Brehm describes a baboon which on being punished by its master never turned on the latter but always attacked anybody else who chanced to be near.

Man, and his subject animals, communicate with each other through sounds, glances, gestures, and touch. The understanding of these signs may demand a process of learning or it may come about spontaneously. There is no exaggeration in the oft-repeated assertion that man and dog understand one another by a glance, or that the ape, particularly the anthropoid ape, is so human in look and gesture that he can at once make himself understood by man. For men themselves do not always require words for mutual comprehension; it is therefore quite conceivable that such comprehension should exist, within limits, between man and the creatures most like him, the anthropoids, or between man and that animal which is capable of attaching itself so affectionately to him, the dog.

Within the limits set by nature it is also possible to communicate with birds. Schjelderup-Ebbe describes the case of the grey parrot. When it wants food or caresses, this bird nestles up to its keeper, hops or dances along its perch, whistles a tune, and utters soft, pleasing, coaxing sounds. If it does not get what it wants it stamps and shrieks until it gains its desire.

Schulz gives an example of the great extent to which animals sometimes learn to understand their masters and respond to their intentions. He hunted zebras and antelopes on horseback in East Africa, and captured them with a lasso. The horse very quickly learns to recognize his rider's intentions, and itself becomes so filled with the excitement of the chase that it occasionally bites the captured zebra. Some antelopes, when hunted, will make a sharp turn in their flight ; the horse of its own accord immediately makes the same turn. Dogs are reported to display similar traits during the chase.

One purpose among others for which dogs are employed in consequence of their versatility is that of guarding live-stock. In this task they behave at each moment as the situation demands : they treat lambs much more gently than sheep. It must here be mentioned that domesticated cranes will shepherd flocks of birds and four-legged beasts exactly like dogs, without having been trained to do so. And a captive agami can lead and keep together a flock of domesticated fowls.

Those species have become domesticated animals, in the strict sense of the word, which are of some definite use to their keeper. As I have said man is unable to create anything that is strictly new by the art of breeding ; he can but transmit variants particularly suited to his purposes from one generation to another by means of appropriate selection and rejection. But since nothing absolutely new can be charmed into existence it is all the more necessary that the breeder should keep his eyes open for novel and favourable morphological, physiological and psychological variants.

o

Pfungst declares that dogs derive from wolves and jackals, not from foxes, and proves that here, too, domestication has brought nothing new into being. Thus he noticed that the rudiments of retrieving show themselves in the play of entirely untrained young wolves.

By consistent selection man has brought some animals to the point of behaving almost as automata under his hand, so that of their own accord they may exert themselves to the utmost in their work. Any peculiarities of behaviour which are the result of training have to be learnt afresh by each generation of animals (hunting hawks, sporting dogs, the *haute école* in the case of horses) ; it is therefore only the ability to learn and not what is learned that is inherited. Many domesticated animals, through their association with men, have entirely lost their original sociological organization into mateships, families, or societies; it is in consequence largely inadmissible to draw conclusions about the behaviour of animals in general from the behaviour of domesticated animals.

It is only races and species capable of adaptation which have been domesticated by man, e.g. horses and asses ; zebras, on the other hand, are hard to tame ; for exhibition purposes it is necessary to place them with ponies which then act as " instructors ". Indian elephants, captured full grown, become friendly with man within a few weeks and do the work demanded of them willingly ; the African elephant, on the other hand, is much less adaptable.

" Domesticated animals " are also to be found in ant and termite states. But it is characteristic of these " domesticated animals " that among themselves they are unsocial or live at the most in loose associations. They either provide their keepers with nutriment in which case they may be called true " cattle ", or they produce a luxury only, namely their exudations, and are then called symphilæ. These latter, together with certain species which serve as " cattle ", are in every respect so completely adapted to their parasitical mode of life that without their hosts they perish ; conversely some ants are entirely dependent upon being nourished by certain kinds of lice.

X HUMAN SOCIOLOGY FROM A BIOLOGICAL STANDPOINT

No matter how we choose to approach the question of the origin of man, this much must be taken as certain, namely that from an anatomical and physiological point of view he belongs to the animal kingdom. Palæontology teaches us that in earlier days men existed of a lower morphological type than the men of to-day; and history shows that man has progressed at least in the sense of attaining more complete knowledge. It is a familiar quarrel whether the difference between the mentality of man and the mentality of animals is one of genus or merely of degree. But the difference between the point of view from which each side appraises the mental characteristics of men and animals is too great to permit the bringing about of any rapid reconciliation between the two divergent opinions. In the course of this essay there have been many instances of characteristics common to both men and animals; instances which make it possible on the ground of psychological data to rank the two together. Nevertheless, it must not be forgotten that men possess certain mental qualities possessed by no animal, and this fact indicates a difference between the two which, in some respects, is fundamental.

The most prominent feature of the greater number of human actions is that the variable factor, V, more or less

completely outweighs the purely instinctive constant factor,
C (*vide* introduction). As instances of actions in which the
instinctive factor preponderates, we may quote sucking in
a newly born infant and the sexual act. But in every action,
even those which at first sight appear purely intellectual,
C and V are indissolubly united. Some things which in men
are governed by tradition (V > C) depend in animals upon
instinct alone (C > V) ; thus in men tradition has to fill
the gap left by the lack of instinctive certainty. The fact
that among men the formula is almost always V > C, and
that V as a rule largely preponderates, explains why in
human societies, schools, courts of justice, parliaments, etc.,
can exist, but not why they actually do exist. Among the
state-building insects, where C on the contrary has so dis-
proportionate a superiority, such institutions cannot occur.
From its earliest moments the newly hatched insect has at
its disposal all the "knowledge" necessary for life. Man has
almost everything to learn by experience, but he inherits
the power to collect experience, and inheritance determines
the range of possible experiences. For man the " norm "
is, then, that nearly all his activities require to be practised,
whereas for insects the " norm " is that almost without
exception no practice is required for the performance of any
activity.

Every species, including the human species, has assigned
to   it   a   definite   morphological,   physiological   and
psychological scope beyond whose limits it cannot go.
Individual variations are possible only within this fixed
scope, the origin of which I shall not now discuss. " Arbitrary
actions " which transcend the limits set for the species never

occur ; every peculiarity of behaviour rests upon a definite physiological and psychological basis. It is, in consequence, altogether erroneous to suppose that human institutions, such as the state, religion, marriage, etc., are purely arbitrary products somewhere and at some time by chance devised by a ruler or a ruling group for their own ease or their own advantage. Were this so, were these institutions not founded upon the inner life of man as a whole, with all its instincts and impulses, they would long ago have disappeared like a passing craze of fashion, and fallen into oblivion. That they have always maintained themselves continuously, even though changing in outward vesture, is the best proof of their natural origin. For men would never arrive at understanding each other even in the simplest matters if the idea to be understood did not rest upon some common universal foundation.

It would be an interesting, though for plain reasons an altogether impossible, experiment to arrange for a number of children to grow up in a state of complete savagery in order to find out what social organizations man is capable of creating without the help of tradition. The outcome of this experiment would naturally vary according to the individuals concerned in it. But it is certain that such isolated human beings would create a community of some kind, and equally mateships and families, in addition to a religion and some form of language ; artistic activities and certain ceremonies would be found among them, festivals would be celebrated, traditional dances would be invented, and so forth. They would pursue theoretical and practical knowledge in some guise or form, however barbarous their chosen methods or procedure might appear to us. (It may, nevertheless, be hinted that possibly our own collective modern wisdom might appear in no better light to some " sovereign spirit ".)

Not every author recognizes with sufficient clearness how firmly all the behaviour of men and animals is rooted in instinct. Thus Whitman denies that those pigeons which form monogamous mateships (and among which occasional infidelities occur) possess a special " instinct of fidelity " ; he argues that we cannot speak of " ethical ideals " in connexion with pigeons, and that the birds hold together only because no opportunity for unfaithfulness occurs. Nevertheless, to this it must be opposed that no lasting social organization—were it merely a colony of brooding pigeons—could possibly be built up on such haphazard foundations. The *sine qua non* of every social organization is that the individuals comprising it shall instinctively react in an appropriate manner to the given milieu, shall adjust themselves to given circumstances. Less essential things may then come to the support of this indispensable factor, e.g. respect for the beaks of other mated pigeons, the claims of nest-building, the necessity for tending the young, etc. Did there not exist in pigeons a certain instinct for monogamy there would still be time for them, in the midst of all their occupations, to indulge in promiscuity.

If we seek to understand clearly the origin of the " ethical ideals " of human beings, we are forced to recognize that they depend upon the whole system of instincts and impulses which man possesses solely in virtue of his being a social creature. Although the outward vesture of these ideals may change from race to race and from time to time, nothing they contain has at any time been arbitrarily contrived by any man ; they may be explained by the roundabout ways of reason, but their source lies in the irrational. If man were an asocial animal it is probable that ethical ideals would not exist at all or would be limited to the relations between male and female and their offspring ; most of the ideals would be purely egoistic.

Among both men and animals a profound conservatism secures the continued existence of an organized society, namely the impulse to maintain what has once become traditional. By this means the social organization, once created, remains in being ; rebellions and riots are invariably followed by some form of social existence. Social beings will always evolve some kind of society ; and this, both among men and many animals, is a graded hierarchy in which one or more individuals assume the part of leader ; the instinct to rule in the superiors is correlated with an instinct of subordination in their inferiors.

Pfungst, Köhler and others point out that in apes the range of interest is never entirely restricted to the immediate necessities of life. The same cause accounts for the irrational, instinctive, insatiable thirst for knowledge in man. This thirst is imperfectly expressed by the proverb " *non scholæ sed vitæ discimus* ". For in the main we seek knowledge neither for school nor life, but because the " daimon " within us compels us to do so. It was not by accident that this proverb was in everyone's mouth, in the age of rationalism. The desire for knowledge in man has its counterpart in a desire to teach and communicate knowledge, of which the root is only to a very minor degree to be found in the pleasure to be derived from a sense of superiority. The desire to teach and the desire to learn are the presuppositions of any comprehensive tradition ; and this, in turn, gives rise to a body of knowledge which increases from generation to generation. Tradition among men has above all this advantage over tradition among animals, namely that it has a cumulative effect, in which speech and technical expedients play a most important part. In my opinion the greatest discovery of the nineteenth century was that of man's unbounded technical inventiveness.

The development of tradition involved, among human beings, a far more intensive cultivation of relations between those united by ties of blood, than is found among animals, where the family frequently disintegrates as soon as the young are full-grown ; and we have no sign that full-grown animals feel themselves more closely bound to one another in virtue of a common ancestry.

The curiosity and energy of captive anthropoid apes are seen to be squandered in purely playful activities. Yet the instincts concerned are exactly similar to those which, more precisely adjusted, underlie the gradual progress made by man in the direction of civilization and culture. If the anthropoid apes landed themselves in an evolutionary blind alley, one of the main reasons was their inability of their own accord to direct their superfluous energies. We find that, in general, the more nearly animals are related to us the closer the resemblance between their instincts and our own, whether these instincts be egoistic, altruistic, or of other kinds. The egoistic instincts, in particular, have a way of appearing less undisguised among men ; but for all that human motives are often fundamentally quite as gross as those of any other mammal, only a whole arsenal of abstract ideas is employed to deck them out in a more pleasing garb.

The playful activities of apes contradict the "law of parsimony" so dear to natural science, according to which every species is endowed only with the abilities and characteristics which are absolutely necessary in the struggle for existence. If we try to apply this principle to the case of man, it becomes clear that his whole existence is one continued refutation of "the law of parsimony"; and we are forced to recognize that side by side with such a principle, if indeed it exists at all, a "principle of extravagance" must also reign not only in the case of men but throughout all animate nature. Phylogenesis in its progress may sometimes make use of the latter principle.

Racial evolution must not be regarded as conditioned by external and fortuitous environmental factors alone; internal factors are always, probably more so than any other, of decisive importance; yet, of these factors, whether they be internal or external, we know absolutely nothing. For instance, it was not merely the fact that the ancestors of man had hands that occasioned the development of man; for in that case why are not all apes men? It is an error to regard the cause of phylogenetic development as so superficial; probably in all cases it goes much deeper.

Man is a creature living in societies. It is most likely that these societies were originally always organized, closed communities. As they develop, societies tend to become less exclusive, and, like the states and large cities of the present

day, acquire in some respects precisely the character
of associations. It is a commonplace that a man may live
most alone in a great town. Thus for some individuals a
large city is nothing more than an association in a milieu
they themselves have created. (Compare what is said
above of the *Paramœcium.*) But since man is a social
animal, in every association links are usually at once
fashioned between its component individuals who thus
become united into societies interrelated in many ways.

I mentioned in my preface that it is idle to ask whether
" in nature " the society or the family is the older type of
companionship. This much may be said : comparing
solitary with social life the former is the lower form ; herd
life exists only among the highest animals. Mateship and
the family on the one hand, and herd life on the other,
rest upon two totally different instincts ; these two forms
may co-exist in one and the same species, as when mateships and families are formed within the herd, or they
may mutually exclude one another, as when a herd each
year divides up into monogamous or polygynous mateships
at the beginning of the breeding season. Among men,
as among many animals, the instinct for conjugal and
family companionship and the herd instinct appear together,
and there is no reason to suppose that among primitive men
the case was different. Until there is proof to the contrary
we may assume, then, that the hordes of the latter, together
with those of his progenitors, always consisted of a number
of single mateships and families. The existence of human
speech is in itself evidence that primitive man was a social
being. All the theories of primitive man living in a state

of idyllic promiscuity gain no support from anything hitherto discovered. If promiscuity, in one form or another, has at any time occurred, it has always been merely as an accessory phenomenon ; closely knit mateships and families have always been (and are to-day) the twin supporters and preservers of the race as a whole and the many individual races.

Men do not possess what earlier authors called "innate ideas ". There is instead a pre-formed basis, C, for ideas, but these only come later. An innate idea of God, gods, and spirits does not exist ; but men of all races possess the impulse, derived from C, to indulge in metaphysical speculations ; the particular form these shall take in any individual is always left to V. There are no innate ideas of particular things (a horse, a tree, etc.) ; their formation during individual development is the work of V ; but the general capacity for conceptual thinking pre-exists in C. But perhaps the instinctive activities of insects are analogous to what in human beings would be called the manifestation of an " innate idea ".

The possibility of religion was given when man began to form ideas on the one hand about his dependence upon his environment, and on the other about the demands made by his own egoistic and social instincts. He objectified the demands of " the inner voice " into gods and goddesses more or less spiritually conceived. A rich growth of imaginative theories entwined themselves around these, and satisfied his need of metaphysical speculation.

Animals also obey an " inner voice ", and " have no choice " when they sacrifice themselves to the rearing of

their young or some other social activity. In itself it would
certainly be " pleasanter " for the bird to eat, to sun itself,
etc., than to build a nest and rear a brood ; but the " inner
voice " enjoins the latter. The animal is guided by its
instincts, and does not ponder over them. Man, in virtue
of the preponderance of V, is forced to make himself clear
as to the moral demands of his inner nature. He recognizes
the moral order fixed for himself and enlarges it into a
moral ordering of the universe ; every race does so in its
own way. If the different species of animals were gifted,
as men are, with a propensity for speculation each would
construct a world order cut to its own pattern, and every
one of these world orders would be valid and " real " within
the circle of individuals for which it was created.

BIBLIOGRAPHY

ALLESCH, G. J. v.: *Bericht über die drei ersten Lebensmonate eines Schimpansen* (Sitz.-Ber. Akad. Wiss. Berlin), 1921.

ALVERDES, F.: *Über Reflexe, Instinkt- und Verstandestätigkeiten* (Zool. Anz., Bd. 60), 1924.

—— *Über vergleichende Soziologie* (Zeitschr. f. Völkerpsychol. u. Soziol., Bd. 1), 1925.

BALDWIN, S. P.: *Adventures in Bird Banding in 1921* (The Auk), 1922.

BALSS, H.: *Über Anpassungen und Symbiose der Paguriden* (Zeitschr. f. Morphol. u. Ökol., Bd. 1), 1924.

BERGER, A.: *In Afrikas Wildkammern als Forscher und Jäger.* 2nd ed. Berlin, 1922.

—— *Über Brunft- und Setzzeit in den Tropen* (Wild u. Hund., 28. Jahrg.), 1922.

BREHMS: *Tierleben*, Bd. 1–13. 4th ed. by v. O. zur Strassen. Leipzig and Vienna, 1912–8.

BUCHNER, P.: *Tier und Pflanze in intrazellularer Symbiose.* Berlin, 1921.

BUTTEL-REEPEN, H. v.: *Die stammesgeschichtliche Entstehung des Bienenstaates.* Leipzig, 1903.

—— *Das Leben und Wesen der Bienen.* Braunschweig, 1915.

DARWIN, Ch.: *Die Abstammung des Menschen.* Übers. v. J. V. Carus. 2nd ed. Stuttgart, 1899.

DEEG, J.: *Über Brunft- und Setzzeit in den Tropen* (Wild und Hund., 28. Jahrg.), 1922.

DEEGENER, P.: *Die Formen der Vergesellschaftung im Tierreiche.* Berlin, 1918.

—— *Soziologische Studien an Raupen und Bemerkungen über Licht- und statischen Sinn* (Arch. f. Naturgesch. 86. Jahrg. Abt. A.), 1920.

—— *Soziologische Beobachtungen an Hyponomeuta cognatellus Hb.* (Biol. Zentralbl., Bd. 42), 1922.

DOFLEIN, F.: *Das Tier als Glied des Naturganzen*—in R. Hesse and F. Doflein, *Tierbau und Tierleben*, Bd. 2. Leipzig and Berlin, 1914.

EIDMANN, H.: *Das Mitteilungsvermögen der Ameisen* (Naturwissensch. Jahrg. 13), 1925.

ESCHERICH, K.: *Die Termiten oder weissen Ameisen.* Leipzig, 1909.

—— *Die Ameise.* 2nd ed. Braunschweig, 1917.

ESPINAS, A. : *Die tierischen Gesellschaften.* Übers. v. W. Schloesser. Braunschweig, 1879.

FOREL, A. : *Le monde social des fourmis.* 5 vols. Geneva, 1921–3.

FRIESE, H. : *Die europäischen Bienen (Apidae).* Berlin and Leipzig, 1923.

FRISCH, K. v. : *Beitrag zur Kenntnis sozialer Instinkte bei solitären Bienen* (Biol. Zentralbl., vol. 38), 1918.

—— *Über die "Sprache" der Bienen* (Zool. Jahrb., Abt. Allg., vol. 40), 1923.

GAETKE, H. : *Die Vogelwarte Helgoland.* Braunschweig, 1891.

GARNER, R. L. : *Die Sprache der Affen.* Übers. v. W. Marshall. Leipzig, 1900.

GEYR v. SCHWEPPENBURG, H. : *Zur Sexualethologie der Stockente* (Journ. f. Ornithol., Bd. 72), 1924.

GIRTANNER, A. : *Aus dem Leben des Alpen-Murmeltiers (Arctomys marmotta L.).* (Zool. Garten, 44. Jahrg.), 1903.

GOETSCH, W. : *Die Abhängigkeit sozialer Insekten vom Nest* (Sitz-Ber. Ges. Morphol. u. Physiol.). Münschen. Jahrg. 34, 1923.

GUENTHER, K. : *Über die " denkenden Tiere "* (Zool. Anz., vol. 52), 1921.

HAECKER, V. : *Der Gesang der Vögel.* Jena, 1900.

HEYDE, K. : *Die Entwicklung der psychischen Fähigkeiten bei Ameisen und ihr Verhalten bei abgeänderten biologischen Bedingungen* (Biol. Zentralbl., vol. 44), 1924.

HUDSON, W. H. : *The Naturalist in La Plata.* 3rd ed. London, 1895.

JACOBI, A. : *Mimikry und verwandte Erscheinungen.* Braunschweig, 1913.

JENNINGS, H. S. : *Das Verhalten der niederen Organismen.* Übers. v. E. Mangold. Leipzig, 1910.

JORDAN, H. : *Vergleichende Physiologie wirbelloser Tiere,* vol. 1. Jena, 1913.

KATZ, D. : *Tierpsychologie und Soziologie des Menschen* (Zeitschr. f. Psychol., vol. 88), 1922.

—— und TOLL, A. : *Die Messung von Charakter- und Begabungsunterschieden bei Tieren (Versuche mit Hühnern)* (Zeitschr. f. Psychol. und Physiol., Abt. 1, vol. 93), 1923.

KOEHLER, W. : *Intelligenzprüfungen an Anthropoiden* (I. Abhandl. Akad. Wiss. Berlin : Phys.-Math. Kl.), 1917.

—— *Zur Psychologie des Schimpansen* (Psychol. Forsch., vol. 1), 1921.
     English trans. of the former *sub tit.* " The Mentality of Apes ", containing the latter—" The Psychology of Chimpanzees " as an Appendix. Kegan Paul & Co. Second (revised) ed., 1927.

KORSCHELT, E. : *Lebensdauer, Altern, und Tod.* 3rd ed. Jena, 1924.

KRIEG, H.: *Studien über Verwilderung bei Tieren und Menschen in Süd-amerika* (Arch. f. Rassen- u. Gesellschaftsbiol., vol. 16), 1925.

KROPOTKIN, P.: *Gegenseitige Hilfe in der Tier- und Menschenwelt.* Übers. v. G. Landauer. Leipzig, 1908.

LUCANUS, F. v.: *Die Rätsel des Vogelzuges.* Langensalza, 1922.

MEISENHEIMER, J.: *Geschlecht und Geschlechter im Tierreiche,* vol. i. Jena, 1921.

MORGAN, C. L.: *Instinkt und Gewohnheit.* Übers. v. M. Semon. Leipzig and Berlin, 1909.

MÜLLER-LYER, F.: *Formen der Ehe, der Familie, und der Verwandtschaft.* München, 1911.

—— *Die Familie.* München, 1912.

MURPHY, R. C.: *The Most Valuable Bird in the World* (Nation. Geogr. Mag., vol. 46), 1924.

NAUMANN'S *Naturgeschichte der Vögel Mitteleuropas.* Herausg. v. C. Hennicke, vols. i-xii. Gera, 1905.

OERTZEN, J. v.: *In Wildnis und Gefangenschaft.* Berlin, 1913.

PECKHAM, G. und E.: *Instinkt und Gewohnheiten der solitären Wespen.* Übers. v. W. Schoenichen. Berlin, 1904.

PFUNGST, O.: *Zur Psychologie der Affen.* Bericht 5. Kongr. f. exper. Psychol. 1912.

—— *Versuche und Beobachtungen an jungen Wölfen.* Bericht 6. Kongr. f: exper. Psychol. 1914.

REICHENOW, E.: *Biologische Beobachtungen an Gorilla und Schimpanse* (Sitz.-Ber. Ges. Naturforsch. Freunde, Jahrg. 1920). Berlin.

RENSCH, B.: *Zur Entstehung der Mimikry der Kuckuckseier* (Journ. f. Ornith., vol. 72), 1924.

ROTHMANN, M. und TEUBER, E.: *Aus der Anthropoidenstation auf Teneriffa I.* (Abhandl. Akad. Wiss.: Phys.-Math. Kl.). Berlin, 1915.

RÜSCHKAMP, F.: *Instinktmodifikationen in einer Ameisen-Adoptions-kolonie* (Zeitschr. f. wiss. Insektenbiol., vol. 19), 1924.

SCHILLINGS, C. G.: *Mit Blitzlicht und Büchse.* Leipzig, 1905.

—— *Der Zauber des Elelescho.* Leipzig, 1906.

SCHJELDERUP-EBBE, Th.: *Beiträge zur Sozialpsychologie des Haushuhns* (Zeitschr. f. Psychol., vol. 88), 1922.

—— *Das Leben der Wildente in der Zeit der Paarung* (Psychol. Forsch., vol. 3), 1923.

—— *Der Graupapagei in der Gefangenschaft* (Psychol. Forsch., vol. 3), 1923.

SCHMID, B.: *Von den Aufgaben der Tierpsychologie* (Abhandl. z. theoret. Biol., H. 8), 1921.

P

210 BIBLIOGRAPHY

SCHROTTKY, C. : *Soziale Gewohnheiten bei solitären Insekten* (Zeitschr. f. wiss. Insektenbiol., vol. 17), 1922.

SCHULZ, C. : *Auf Grosztierfang für Hagenbeck.* 3rd ed. Dresden, 1922.

SCHUSTER, L. : *Brunft- und Setzzeit des Wildes in den Tropen* (Wild u. Hund., 29. Jahrg.), 1923.

SOKOLOWSKY, A. : *Zur Frage des Geisteslebens der Menschenaffen* (Med. Klinik, Jahrg 5), 1909.

STRESEMANN, E. : *Über gemischte Vogelschwärme* (Verhandl. d. Ornithol. Ges. Bayern, vol. 13), 1917.

THURNWALD, R. : *Psychologie des primitiven Menschen*—in G. Kafka, *Handbuch. d. vgl. Psychologie*, Bd. I, Abt. 2, 1922.

—— *Zur Kritik der Gesellschaftsbiologie* (Arch. f. Sozialwiss., vol. 52), 1924.

VOLZ, W. : *Im Dämmer des Rimba.* Breslau, 1921.

WASMANN, E. : *Die psychischen Fähigkeiten der Ameisen.* 2nd ed. 1909.

—— *Die Gastpflege der Ameisen* (Abhandl. z. theoret. Biol., H. 3), 1920.

—— *Eine interessante Instinktregulation bei Ameisen (Lasius mixtus Nyl.)* (Atti R. Acc. Lincei Rend. Roma. 76), 1923.

—— *Die Ameisenmimikry* (Abhandl. z. theoret. Biol., H. 19), 1925.

WHEELER, W. M. : *Ants.* New York, 1910.

—— *Social Life among the Insects.* New York, 1924.

WHITMAN, Ch. : *The Behavior of Pigeons.* Ed. by H. A. Carr. Carnegie Inst. Washington. Publ. 257. Vol. 3. 1919.

YERKES, R. M. : *The Instincts, Habits, and Reactions of the Frog* (Psychol. Review. Monograph. Suppl., vol. 4). 1903.

—— *The Mental Life of Monkeys and Apes* (Behavior Monographs, vol. 3), 1916.

ZIEGLER, H. E. : *Tierstaaten und Tiergesellschaften* (Handwörterbuch d. Naturwiss., vol. 9), 1913.

—— *Die Urformen der Ehe und des Eigentums* (Mitt. d. Ges. f. Tierpsych., N.F. Nr. 5), 1924.

INDEX

Adoption, 62, 73, 102, 135
Adornment, 155
Agami, 131
Alcippe, 37
Alligator, 68, 134
Alytes obstetricans, 66 ; and promiscuity, 18
Amblyornis, 149
Amia, 67
Ammodytes, 130
Amphibians, 68, 32, 42
Antelopes, 33, 36, 64, 72, 77, 81, 150, 167, 193 ; Oryx, 38 ; N. American, 161 ; Peruvian Pronghorned, 181 ; Saiga, 77, 122
Anergates, 99
Animal societies, 2 ; sociology, 1
Antennæ language, 102, 176
Antilocapra, American, 77
Ants, 1, 142 ; battle fury among, 98 ; building and brood-tending of, 110 ; dependent queens among, 92 ; nuptial flight of, 91 ; queens, 91 ; weaver, 93
Apes, 43, 47, 72, 113, 134, 161, 162, 165, 192
Apes, anthropoid, 3
Ape code, 172 ; greetings, 173 ; language, 171 ; play of, 136 ; societies, 58
Appearance, and psychical condition, 66
Arius, 67
Arthropods, 67
Asses, Asiatic wild, 46 ; Nubian, wild, 46
Associations, 4, 10, 21, 22, 37, 95, 99, 195
Atta, 97 ; morphological polymorphism of, 91
Auks, 53

Baboons, 59, 82, 119, 137 ; Arabian, 112 ; Gelada, 82 ; Hamadryas, 82

Bachelor herds, 40, 72. 79
Bantin, 72
Bats, 79, 159
Bears, 33
Beavers, 38, 77, 118, 137
Bee bread, 88
Bee-eaters, 53
Bees, 21 ; bumble, 142 ; isolated, 110 ; Trumpeter, 86 ; Queen, rearing of, 89
Beetles, 31 ; apothecary (*Ateuchus sacer*), 163 ; bark, 34 ; burying (*Necrophorus*) in associations, 14 ; dung, *Minotaurus typhœus*, 31 ; lamellicorn *Ateuchus sacer*, 31 ; pairing more than once, 18 ; stag, male, 145 ; wood-boring *Passalides*, 31, 60, 158
Betta, 145
Biological meaning, 9
Bisons, 7 ; female (*Bos bonasus*), 79 ; steers, 146 ; N. American, 27
Black game, 28, 37 ; cock, 147
Bonellia, 37
Bouquetins, 78
Bowerbird male, 149
Brazilian anis (*Crotophaga ani*), 57
Breeding societies, 20
Budgerigar, 139
Buffaloes, 2, 72, 79, 122 ; Indian, 35
Building instinct in ants, 93
Bullfinches, 117
Butterflies, 20, 21, 130 ; social tendencies in, 22

Cachalots, 71
Callionimus lyra, 18
Callithrix, 52, 65
Cannibalism, 138
Capercaillies, 28, 37, 147
Copris, 68
Care of Young by Male, 64
Carp, small (*Rhodeus amarus*), 32
Castes, 24, 84

214 INDEX

For Product Safety Concerns and Information please contact our EU
representative GPSR@taylorandfrancis.com
Taylor & Francis Verlag GmbH, Kaufingerstraße 24, 80331 München, Germany

www.ingramcontent.com/pod-product-compliance
Ingram Content Group UK Ltd.
Pitfield, Milton Keynes, MK11 3LW, UK
UKHW021426080625
459435UK00011B/169